# Skin Care: Clear & Simple

Ligaya H. Buchbinder, M.D.

*A leading dermatologist guides you through your common skin, hair, and nail problems and gives you helpful advice on their care.*

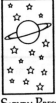

SATURN PRESS

I. Skin Care: Clear & Simple
Copyright © 1997 by Ligaya H. Buchbinder, M.D.
First Edition

Cataloging in Publication Data available from Library of Congress.

Library of Congress Catalog Card Number: 96-93067
International Standard Book Number: 1-885843-05-4

Printed in the United States of America

Cover design by Lightbourne Images, Inc.

Published by:
Saturn Press, Inc.
17639 Foxborough Lane
Boca Raton, FL 33496

Skin Care: Clear & Simple is not intended as a substitute for the medical advice of a physician.

Readers should consult with their physicians/dermatologists regarding any skin care disorders or treatments.

# Dedication

*For my husband, Charles, and my truly great children, Aaron and Lana.*
*For my mother, Consejo, and my late father, Fernando, who devoted their lives to their children's education. They were public school teachers who through self-sacrifice and strong determination provided for their three children to attend medical school and become physicians.*

*Thank you, Dad. I am living your dream.*

# Acknowledgments

I would like to express my sincerest gratitude to my patient, Jean Stanley. She came to my office one day and asked me, "Doctor, why don't you write a book on skin care? I was unable to find a good updated book on this subject written by a dermatologist for the layman. I myself have written two published books, and I will help you however I can." I promised her that I would think about it.

I came home that day and told my husband, "I think I will write a book on skin care." He knew that once I declared my intention, a book would materialize. A dermatologist himself, he offered to edit the book for me.

We took off for Bangkok two weeks later for our much-awaited R&R. On our way home, I asked Dr. Martin Luther King III who was sitting beside me on the plane from San Francisco to autograph my half-finished manuscript which he graciously did.

I am also grateful to Drs. Marc and Kathy Levinson for making the publication of this book a reality and to my editor, Erica Orloff, who regarded this book as her personal skin care adviser. She asked all the questions that she wants answered by the expert and I am delighted to answer them in this book.

I think of Jean, Kathy, Erica, and myself as the four winds who blew to burn the phoenix. Jean is the west wind who started to blow, Kathy is the south wind who opened its gust, Erica is the east wind who twisted and turned and I am the north wind who blew and blew to consume the phoenix into its ashes. We sat, we waited, and we saw this phoenix (book) rise from its ashes.

# Preface

Your skin, hair, and nails comprise the outermost covering of your body. Every year, billions of dollars are spent on cosmetics and skin care products. Several more billions are spent on hair and nail care, clothing, hair fashion, and nail fashion. Why all this spending? Simple answer — everyone wants to look good.

Since our skin, hair, and nails create our first physical impression to the world, we will focus on their care and beauty. A basic understanding of these components will help us know how to take care of what nature gave us. In this book, we will also explore how to enhance what we naturally have. The tangible rewards for proper skin, hair, and nail care will include trouble-free skin and improved hair and nail appearance which saves us a lot of anguish and money. After all, it is easier and less expensive to enhance instead of completely redoing or covering up. Because nature provided us with this cover, why not try to understand it? First impressions are lasting and our skin, hair, and nails create our first impressions to the world.

There is nothing better than good basic skin care, but magazines, television shows, commercials, and cosmetic ads are full of complicated and sometimes contradictory advice. Actually, it is really very easy and inexpensive. If you are willing to give it a try, this book will give you simple and easy ideas and hopefully convince you that your skin is not bad after all. A simple routine is all you need to face the world with your own natural beauty!

I have drawers full of cosmetics and countertops full of this and that, but guess what? Every morning I get in the shower, wash my face with soap and water, shampoo and condition my hair, dry myself, apply a moisturizer from my face down to my feet, dab a little blush on, apply my favorite color lipstick, and I'm ready to put on my clothes and go to work. Off I go. This is me at my best!

Come join me on a journey from skin to self as we go through the pages of this book. In reading through these chapters, you and I will get acquainted on three different levels. You will read my mind, hear my heartbeat, and touch my spirit. Writing this book is a personal journey for me because I wrote in this book what I learned, thought, practiced, and loved. My father always taught me to use my common sense. Common sense is indeed necessary to survive, but add a touch of courage and a sprinkle of love — then life is certainly worth living!

# Contents

# Chapter 1

# The Skin: Your Unique First Impression

*Mirror, mirror on the wall, who is the fairest of us all?*
*Thou art the fairest since thou beholdest.*

Your skin is your showcase to the world, as well as your security blanket from the world. The skin serves as our external covering and protects our body from excessive heat and water loss. It also helps regulate our body temperature. The outermost wrapper of our internal organs, it presents our body as a gift to the world. A vital element of our identity, the skin sets us apart from other individuals. Nature brilliantly creates individual human beings! No two skins are alike, not even among identical twins.

How do we set the standard for good skin? All individuals are born with their own set of genes that pretty much determines how they are supposed to look as they grow up. Isn't it logical to set this genetic makeup as the relative norm for each individual? We grow up and get used to what we basically own. We also get accustomed to what we see in the mirror every day and I refer to this as genetic sensitization. Therefore, every person's skin is unique because every individual is unique.

All individuals are born to this planet earth, and we all live and interact with each other. Who determines what is normal or abnormal? Who determines what is good and what is bad? Did we all agree on a certain standard?

What is normal skin to the individual? Since there are individual, familial, and racial genetic differences, normal skin is quite relative when we consider the total picture. Normal skin can be viewed in two perspectives. One perspective is based on the changes that an individual's skin undergoes in relation to his or her genetically predetermined characteristics. The second perspective is based on the changes that an individual's skin undergoes in relation to the skin genetics of the general population. What is normal skin to the dermatologist? There are dermatology books based on the genetics of the individual as well as the genetics of the society as a whole. The dermatologist is basically concerned with what is healthy skin and what is unhealthy skin. Healthy skin is normal skin and unhealthy skin is a condition out of balance. Health is the opposite of disease. Healthy skin is the state of skin that does not cause an individual "dis-ease."

Skin "dis-ease," generally, is what brings a patient to the dermatologist. The dermatologist's job is to determine whether the patient's complaint is a pathological disease or not. We define a pathological skin disease as a skin disorder which is recognized as a disease entity in the medical literature. In the case of a pathological skin disease, the dermatologist usually gives the patient a prescription and offers advice regarding the disease. If the dermatologist determines that the problem is not a pathological skin disease, it is the greater job of the dermatologist to cure the patient of this "dis-ease." The dermatologist has the obligation to enlighten the patient regarding his or her condition with the hope that the patient walks out of the office relieved of the dis-ease and restored to a healthy state.

The following pages of this book will discuss common skin diseases along with straightforward skin care. This dermatologist wishes to enlighten you to some of your skin "dis-eases" and hopefully cure them. I want each and every one of my readers to look his or her best.

# Part I _____
## Common Skin Problems

# Chapter 2

# Dry Skin: Restoring Your Skin's Luster

Dry skin is one of the most common causes of non-specific itching. Our skin naturally loses its surface moisture from evaporation. Dry skin also is an important cause of skin luster loss.

Our skin is constantly exposed to the environment. Therefore, it is important to protect our skin from drying out. A simple method to accomplish this is by regular use of a skin moisturizer to seal in the moisture on the skin surface especially after a shower or bath. Moisturizers, made up of different compounds, seal in the water molecules on the skin's surface. Certain moisturizers accomplish this better than others.

There are a multitude of skin moisturizers or emollients available in drug stores, supermarkets, and at cosmetic counters. If you are confused by the many choices, you are not alone. As a dermatologist, I am often asked which one is the best. Some have a thicker consistency than others. Moisturizers also contain many different ingredients that vary from product to product. Some claim all-natural or herbal ingredients. Vitamin E, fruit acids, fragrances, lanolin — the list of ingredients can go on and on. Moisturizers also vary in their prices, from a couple of dollars for a supermarket brand to $80, $90 or more for top designer labels.

Normal, non-problematic skin will probably do well with the majority of the moisturizers available on the market. Individual preference, however, is important in choosing a moisturizer. Some are more cosmetically elegant to the feel compared to others. Dermatologists have their favorite moisturizers that they recommend. A dermatologist's store room is usually filled with moisturizers from A to Z. I, personally, try most of the products promoted by the manufacturers and I pick a handful that I know from training and experience are better than the rest.

Moisturizers also are tested for comedogenicity, which means their tendency to bring about whiteheads or blackheads. I recommend a moisturizer that seals in moisture but does not block the skin pores, otherwise, we end up with acne-like breakouts caused by the plugging of the pores (refer to the chapter on Acne). Try to choose moisturizers labeled non-comedogenic.

More expensive moisturizers are not necessarily better. It is important to read the labels of moisturizers. One important ingredient that I advise the acne-prone to avoid is any form of oil, such as lanolin, petrolatum or mineral oil, which are common moisturizer ingredients. Lanolin is also best avoided by individuals who have a history of eczema because these individuals may be sensitive to lanolin.

It is smart to try any new product on a small area first. Try to ask for a tester if you may. Bear in mind that testing does not mean one-time application. A skin reaction usually occurs after using a new product over a period of days, weeks, or even months.

There are two types of skin allergic reaction: immediate and delayed allergic reactions. There is also another type of skin reaction referred to as an irritant reaction and this usually occurs within a short period of repeated applications. A delayed reaction may develop over a period of days to months. Therefore, short-term testing will expose the immediate reaction and the irritant reaction but may miss the delayed reaction.

Alpha hydroxy acids (AHAs) utilized in lower concentrations are incorporated as active components of many moisturizers on the

---

### WHAT TO LOOK FOR IN A GOOD MOISTURIZER

Non-comedogenic on the label
Try an AHA-containing moisturizer if the regular brands are not
   sufficient
No fragrance if you have sensitive skin
Remember — apply your moisturizer twice a day, preferably once
   after a shower or bath

---

market today. AHAs are mild acids derived from fruits and other natural substances. They are also all the rage at cosmetic counters and in fashion magazines. AHAs make up good moisturizers. However, certain individuals may be sensitive to this ingredient and the most common problem that I see in my office related to this is an irritant skin reaction. AHAs utilized in higher concentrations cause skin exfoliation, thus causing skin to peel. Under the guidance of a properly trained skin care professional, this can be helpful, inducing younger looking skin. However, it is important to exercise healthy caution.

One of the most common causes of wrinkling is dry skin. Part of the problem in fine wrinkling around our eyes is dry skin. Eye creams serve as moisturizers to the delicate skin surrounding the eye. However, I do not recommend putting AHAs on the soft and delicate skin around the eyes. This does not necessarily mean you need an expensive eye cream. Sometimes a simple non-AHA moisturizer will do. Now you can see why I spent much of Chapter 1 talking about each of us as individuals with skin "uniqueness." I cannot wave a magic wand and say any one product is universally perfect for all skin types, all those with dry skin, or all those with acne. Instead, in this book, you and I will take this journey together and find precisely what will work for you.

Now, back to moisturizers. . . . . The skin creates a tough barrier for absorption of chemicals or organic substances. Therefore, most of the substances that we apply on the surface of the skin basically remains on the surface. The more effective moisturizers are able to bind with the organic molecules of the skin, thus creating a smooth interface. Skin constantly sheds, however, so even the strongest bonds are eventually lost due to shedding. This means that moisturizing should be periodically repeated in order to maintain its desired effect. I recommend moisturizing twice a day. Every day. Your skin will thank you for it by feeling softer and looking more youthful!

# Chapter 3

# Acne: Banish Your Blemishes

Joan, a healthy, pretty 14-year-old girl, came to my office for her first dermatology appointment. Despite eating a healthy diet and careful cleansing, Joan had acne covering most of her face. Emotionally, this caused her a great deal of pain and she was hopeful that I could help her. I first explained what acne was and then set about finding a cleansing regime and a medication to bring her skin under control.

Acne is a very common skin problem that often brings in a patient, like Joan, for the first time to the dermatologist's office. Acne, a follicular occlusion disorder, means that pores which are openings of the hair to the skin surface are clogged. The hair follicle has an oil gland attached to it and is lined by skin cells. In the normal state, sebum or oil and dead skin cells are shed out of these pores without hindrance. However, in acne these pores are clogged with dead skin cells, causing an occlusion of the hair follicle. Like a clogged pipe, a build-up of sebum and dead skin cells results and whiteheads or blackheads are formed. With further build-up of sebum and dead skin cells, the hair follicle balloons and results in a pimple. Within this pimple, bacteria proliferates. The pimple may continue to swell and rupture. This is referred to as cystic acne — the most scarring form of this skin disease.

Mild to moderate acne may not leave a scar if treated in time. Most of the scarring resulting from mild to moderate acne is caused by picking at the pimples. Picking causes more damage to the skin on top of the acne because the nails cause irregular breaks to the skin surface. The deeper you pick, the higher the likelihood of a scar. The harder you squeeze, the more likely you will end up with skin discoloration.

Do certain types of food cause acne? No strong scientific evidence exists suggesting any particular food causes acne. However, if a particular food repeatedly seems to cause your skin to break out, it will be wise for you to stay away from it. In addition, eating fruits and vegetables rich in vitamins and minerals and drinking sufficient amounts of water help in maintaining healthy skin. I recommend drinking at least eight 8-ounce glasses of water a day. My personal philosophy is that a balanced diet is important in maintaining healthy skin, hair, and nails.

Let me also dispel a myth here. Acne is not contagious and may arise despite good cleanliness. However, it may occur within a family with a history of acne.

I usually recommend washing the face twice a day (morning and evening) using regular soap and water. Soaping is done with bare hands after thoroughly wetting the face with tepid water. After rinsing, pat dry with a clean cotton towel. Acne does not disappear by scrubbing your face. In fact, I do not recommend scrubbing the face because scrubbing causes additional physical harm to the delicate skin. The application of mild exfoliant creams or lotions containing ascorbic acid (vitamin C) or AHA may improve acne-prone skin.

Common treatments for acne include benzoyl peroxide, azelaic acid (Azelex®), tretinoin (Retin-A®), adapalene (Differin®, a new generation of topical retinoid analog), and topical and oral antibiotics. You may choose to try the over-the-counter preparations prior to seeking expert help. Benzoyl peroxide 5% is available over-the-counter for application to acne breakouts. This is usually applied

---

### ACNE DO'S AND DON'T'S

**Do**

Eat a healthy balanced diet
Drink eight 8-ounce glasses of water daily
Wash your face twice a day, patting gently dry
Try a 5% benzoyl peroxide gel, applied a half hour after washing
Try a 2% to 3% salicylic acid soap bar, 5% to 10% benzoyl peroxide
  bar/liquid wash, or an AHA wash
Try a formulation with ascorbic acid or AHA

**Don't**

Scrub your face
Pick at your pimples
Delay seeking treatment for severe cystic acne

---

twice a day and I recommend waiting at least a half hour after washing the face prior to its application to avoid skin irritation. Some individuals, however, are sensitive to benzoyl peroxide. Skin irritation or burning may occur in this situation. Testing a small area first, over several days of applying the medication to this same area, may help determine whether this treatment is suited to you. Special cleansers which you may try if regular soap is not suited to your skin are: glycolic acid wash, 2% salicylic acid soap bar (Stiefel®), and 5% benzoyl peroxide wash (liquid or bar). If you have the supersensitive skin type, you may use the soap-free cleansers available today (for example, Cetaphil® Gentle Skin Cleanser, Aquanil® Lotion). Soap-free cleansers usually contain a combination of sodium lauryl sulfate, purified water, cetyl alcohol, benzyl alcohol and strearyl alcohol and may cost anywhere from a few dollars to over ten dollars. I advise you to use the more reasonably priced ones because they work just as well.

There is a definite hormonal correlation with acne. Increased amounts of androgen hormones, testosterone, and progesterone increase the activity of sebaceous glands, thus causing or exacerbating acne. Estrogen decreases the activity of sebaceous glands, thereby

ð

### Ligaya On . . . Beauty Inside and Out

*The gentle rush of blood from a smile creates an instant healthy*
*shine on your face. Be still and pay attention . . . . A tingle on your*
*skin occurs, then you feel the warmth in your heart.*

possibly improving acne. There may be premenstrual exacerbation
of acne as well as acne flare-ups at certain stages of pregnancy due to
changes in hormonal levels within our system during these periods.

More severe cases of adult acne are usually treated with oral
antibiotics like tetracycline in addition to topical treatment. Nowadays, even the most severe form of cystic acne can be treated. Seek
early help from a dermatologist or physician if the over-the-counter
remedies that you have tried are not working. A lifetime of permanent scars from acne can be avoided.

## Dr. Ligaya Buchbinder's Favorite
## Acne Regimen

- ð Wash in the morning and evening with 2% salicylic acid
  soap bar (Stiefel®) and cool to tepid water, using your hands.
- ð Pat dry with clean cotton towel.
- ð Apply ascorbyl palmitate with DEA® complex eye cream
  formulation (C-Esta® Eye Cream) — no need for a prescription — to entire face. DEA® complex allows skin
  absorption of the fat soluble form of vitamin C. C-Esta®
  Eye Cream is sometimes available through dermatologists or fine salons or spas or through the manufacturer,
  Jan Marini Skin Research, Inc., San Jose, California.
  Apply sparingly using your fingertip. I prefer the eye
  cream because it is non-comedogenic, non-irritating, and
  quite effective. Apply both morning and night.
- ð Apply adapalene gel (Differin® Gel) or Retin-A Micro™
  (a new formulation of tretinoin 0.1% gel which is less
  irritating to the skin). Apply to acne-prone areas every
  night or every other night.

- You may use sunscreen, moisturizer, powder, water-based foundation, or water-based make-up over C-Esta® Eye Cream, but make sure you wait for it to dry for a few minutes prior to application.
- A short course of antibiotics by mouth (for example, tetracycline, doxycycline, minocycline, cephalosporin, or ampicillin). You need a prescription for these. I recommend the prescription when my patients are erupting with pustules and/or cysts.

My regimen applies to anyone not sensitive to the listed products.

# Chapter 4

# Wrinkling and the Aging Skin: Is There a Fountain of Youth?

Preventing wrinkling and repairing aging skin are two of the most common reasons I see patients nowadays. Years of sunbathing before we knew better have left many of us with prematurely wrinkled skin. And wrinkles are one of the first tell-tale signs of our aging process. People have very mixed emotions about accepting those crow's feet and skin wrinkles. Our culture is very youth oriented. Wrinkles that might be revered in China as associated with wisdom are often dreaded here in the United States.

Natural wrinkling occurs on the lines of our facial expression. However, additional wrinkling occurs with sun damage and the natural process of aging. In sun-damaged skin, there is an increased ratio of cross-linked elastic fibers to collagen. The elastic material appears to replace collagen in the upper part of the dermis (the second layer of the skin beneath the epidermis).

Decreasing skin elasticity leads to wrinkling. Some individuals are genetically more prone to wrinkling compared to others. Ultra-

ᴥ

### Ligaya On . . . The Fountain of Youth

*When I do my Hatha yoga every morning, I notice how my total being can get misaligned from the previous day. I feel very fortunate that Hatha yoga enables me to align and integrate my body, mind, and spirit and start my day fresh from my center. The coordination of breathing, muscular tension and relaxation, balance, and concentration is the crux of Hatha yoga. You cannot help but be completely present in the moment in order to perform the ultimate Hatha yoga. To live in the present moment is the key to enlightenment according to the Zen masters. The memories of the past are now and the dreams of the future are forged now. Do not focus your attention on the past or wander into the future. Pay attention to all the details of now and live this present moment. All things will fall into place and your dreams will be realized. This means that you are creating your future now. Sounds easy, but it is quite a challenge. I am trying. It works! Since I had been practicing Hatha yoga, one universal comment that I get from my friends, patients, and acquaintances is this: "You look so much younger! What are you doing?" I may not have found the fountain of youth, but I am close to certain that I have slowed my aging process.*

violet light exposure is also a very important factor in wrinkling of the skin.

Ultraviolet light has proven to do far-reaching damage to the elastic fibers of the skin. It causes clumping and disintegration of these fibers. This damage is permanent. Skin loosens up like a rubber band left out in the sun too long. It does not recoil back in shape! Because of this loss of substance and loss of elasticity, easy bruising and tearing of the skin also results.

Creams, lotions, and washes with claims of reducing wrinkling predominate the cosmetic counters. The three top active substances highly sought by the public are tretinoin (Renova®, Retin A®) which is a derivative of vitamin A (a prescription is necessary), AHAs, and the newest in the market is ascorbic acid or vitamin C.

Renova® is supposed to demonstrate effectiveness and low incidence of skin irritation, unlike Retin-A® which can cause a significant amount of skin irritancy. I find Renova® not ideal for acne because of its oily base.

Retinoids (vitamin A derivatives) and ascorbic acid have been shown to inhibit skin tumor formation. Ascorbic acid has also been shown to stimulate collagen synthesis.[11,15] Ascorbic acid does not act as a sunscreen but has photo-protective qualities.[12] Vitamin C has to be provided by diet in humans because it is not made by the body. The amount of vitamin C that is delivered to the skin and other tissues is limited when vitamin C is ingested. Therefore, we turn to topical applications of vitamin C in the form of L-ascorbic acid to penetrate the skin's surface and travel to the inner layers where collagen synthesis occurs when applied in a precise formulation and pH level. Topical L-ascorbic acid is quickly absorbed by skin and will remain in the body at maximum effectiveness for up to three days. Ascorbyl palmitate, the lipid soluble form of vitamin C, is normally not absorbed by the skin unless formulated with the proper vehicle to facilitate its absorption (like the DEA Complex® in C-Esta® Eye Cream). With its neutral pH, C-Esta® is normally not irritating to the skin. A moisturizer can be applied after application of a vitamin C formulation on the skin. In general, formulations containing ascorbic acid may be used in conjunction with retinoids or AHAs. Word of caution: Consult your doctor or skin care professional to be certain. There is some variation depending on the particular ascorbic acid formulation that you are using. Some formulations of ascorbic acid may suit your skin better than others.

AHAs in higher concentration are primarily skin exfoliants. They predominantly work on the outer layer of the skin causing the top layer of the skin to peel off to reveal the new cells underneath.

At this point, I have tried tretinoin (Retin-A®, Renova®), AHAs, and vitamin C preparations (C-Esta®, Cellex-C®, Citrix®). I tend to be partial to the beneficial effects of vitamin C as seen on my skin, considering the relatively short amount of time that I have used it so far, compared to the other products. My skin feels smoother, shinier, more even in coloration and has lesser acne breakouts and whitehead formation. One has to be very careful in choosing a product containing any of these active ingredients because one preparation may be

> **WHAT ARE COMMON AHAS?**
>
> Glycolic acid
> Lactic acid
> Mandelic acid
> Benzilic acid

comedogenic compared to another. Depending on your skin type, one preparation of the same product may be more suited for you compared to another. For example, I tried a solution and a cream containing vitamin C made by the same company. I found that the solution made me break out with whiteheads but the cream provided all the beneficial effects of vitamin C that I mentioned above, without the breakout effects. Tretinoin (Retin-A®) did improve my acne, but I am quite bothered by the irritancy that it caused on my skin as well as the darkening on my upper lip and cheeks especially when I am out in the sun, despite my regular use of sunscreens. Renova® is certainly less irritating than Retin-A®, but I broke out most likely because of the oil base of this formulation. Alpha hydroxy acids (AHAs) are a group encompassing a variety of active substances which commonly includes glycolic acid, lactic acid, mandelic acid, and benzilic acid. The bioavailability of free acid determines the efficacy of an AHA product and not necessarily the declared concentration on the label.[18]

Cosmetic procedures are available to improve the appearance of a wrinkled face. This includes face lifts, forehead lifts, collagen injections, fat injections, laser surgery, temporary paralysis of the nerve causing the deep furrows on the middle of the forehead (a new procedure) and chemical peels (refer to Questions and Answers, pp. 123–125). You should discuss these options with a cosmetic surgeon and ask for his or her expert advice as to what is suited for your particular situation. The success of these procedures depends highly on the skill of the surgeon and the proper preparation and care of the patient before, during, and after surgery. Side effects and realistic expectations should be clearly discussed and understood. (See Question and Answer section for more in-depth discussion of this.)

How does one prevent sun-induced wrinkling? I recommend the use of a moisturizer with at least an SPF 15 on a daily basis, even with normal daily activity. One can also use make-up with SPF 15. When one engages in sports or is going swimming, I recommend the water-resistant sunscreens with components that offer protection from UVA and UVB (refer to the Questions and Answers, pp. 137–141). You may try using vitamin C and/or retinoid formulations. Word of caution: Be sure to ask your physician or dermatologist prior to using the two formulations at the same time.

Retinoids and vitamin C have been shown to improve some amount of superficial sun damage when used over an extended period, assuming that the person is extremely careful to not add any further sun damage. I am not convinced that AHAs in lower concentrations (as incorporated in moisturizers) improve sun-damaged skin. Short of a chemical peel which is usually performed by some dermatologists and plastic surgeons (I discuss in-depth in Questions and Answers), 5-fluoro uracil (Efudex®) is prescribed under strict supervision by a dermatologist for removal of precancerous growths and improvement of sun-damaged skin. This is usually applied on the skin by the patient for a period of 3 to 4 weeks for optimum results. Extensive studies have now confirmed the remarkable effectiveness of

---

## PROTECTING YOUR SKIN DO'S AND DON'T'S

### Do

Wear an SPF 15 sunscreen every day
If you wear make-up, choose foundation with an SPF 15
Wear a hat when out in the sun for sports or beach fun
Wear sunglasses that block UVB and UVA rays
Reapply sunscreen if out in the sun for long periods of time or if in the water for extended periods of time

### Don't

Sunbathe!!
Wear oils and other tan-inducing lotions to the beach

the drug beta carotene in improving the tolerance of patients suffering from a photosensitive disorder called porphyria to sun exposure.[4]
Whether beta carotene is effective in affording photoprotection to the
general population is not clearly answered.

## What's New on the Horizon?

- Vitamin C incorporated in creams and lotions has prom-
  ising potential for preventing premature aging of the skin
  (for example, C-Esta®, Cellex-C®).
- Adapalene (Differin Gel® — you need a prescription) is
  the newest generation of retinoid analog now out in the
  market.
- AHAs.
- Ascorbic acid — the precise formulation, concentration,
  and pH affects its efficacy on the skin. Cellex-C® contains L-ascorbic acid which is the water soluble form of
  vitamin C. C-Esta® contains ascorbyl palmitate in a
  DEA® complex vehicle.
- Bentoquatam 5% (IvyBlock®) is a new drug approved by
  the FDA to protect the skin from poison ivy, oak, or
  sumac. I cannot comment on its efficacy as a protective
  barrier at this time.
- Tretinoin is available in a less irritating formulation
  (Renova®) for wrinkling and sun-damaged skin.
- Retin-A Micro™ is the new formulation of tretinoin 0.1%
  gel which is less irritating to the skin for the treatment of
  acne.

# Chapter 5

# Rosacea: Remedying Your Redness

B arbara, a 45-year-old travel executive, came to my office complaining of redness and flushing on her face. She described her skin tone as "ruddy" and said she had to wear heavy concealer and make-up just to get an even skin tone. In the heat of South Florida, the heavy make-up was unpleasant for her to have to put on and wear every day, and she was finally seeking treatment for her redness. After examining Barbara and listening to her symptoms, I played detective. Did the redness ever worsen? With sun exposure? What about if Barbara ate hot, spicy foods? After her morning cup of coffee? A few more detective questions and I found the culprit and made my diagnosis: rosacea.

Rosacea is a skin disorder usually occurring in middle-aged to older persons. It usually occurs on the face and is characterized by redness, prominent blood vessels visible on the skin surface, enlarged oil glands, and acne-like breakouts. Rosacea may also affect the eyes, neck, scalp, and upper chest. In severe cases of rosacea, the nose may grow larger. This is caused by the enlargement of the soft tissues under the skin on the oil-gland rich nose.

---

## ROSACEA DO'S AND DON'T'S

### Do

Wear an SPF 15 sunscreen every day — even if you are not headed
    for the beach!
Wear a hat in warmer climates to protect your face even further from
    the sun
Use a mild, non-irritating cleanser
Avoid the following:
      caffeine
      chocolate
      heavy spices like red pepper and cayenne pepper
      alcohol
      tomatoes
Stay cool

### Don't

Stay out in the sun too long even with a sunscreen on
Scrub your skin
Use grainy exfoliators

---

Patients suffering with rosacea may notice sudden increased redness of the cheeks and nose during periods of heightened emotions, and during or after exercise, sun exposure, drinking alcohol, caffeine, or eating certain foods like tomatoes and spices.

There are some myths we can dispel about rosacea. It is not contagious but may run in the family. You must have a tendency for rosacea in order to suffer an exacerbation. Another myth debunked: Rosacea is not a disease of alcoholics.

Common treatments for rosacea include the use of mild skin cleansers and avoiding foods that are known to exacerbate rosacea. These include caffeine, chocolate, spices, alcohol, and tomatoes. Sun protection using sunscreens with an SPF 15 (sun protection factor) or higher and the use of physical protection from the sun like a hat or an umbrella is highly recommended. In tropical countries, the use of an umbrella for sun protection is a common and wise custom.

A note of caution: If rosacea is persistent, the use of topical or oral antibiotics is recommended. You should not wait to suffer the irreversible consequences of rosacea like an enlarged nose. See your dermatologist or physician. Something can be done before it is too late.

☙

## Ligaya On . . . The Serenity of Silence

*The mind needs a "time out," even for 15 minutes a day when we are awake. This practice enables us to listen to the sound of silence — perhaps a message from our higher mind. It is quite difficult to still the mind amidst a multitude of external and internal chatter. Helpful hint: Focus your attention on your breath. Take a few abdominal breaths. Pay complete attention to the air coming in and going out of your nose. Do this practice at any time during your waking hours, either while standing or walking. When you feel tense or anxious, STOP! Focus your full attention on your breath. Note the difference after a few breaths. You can extend this practice for longer periods daily and you will notice a definite improvement in your well-being. Your skin reflects the state of your being. Pay attention and you will notice what I am talking about. You will frown less, thus lessening your frown lines. You will break out less. You will itch less. Best of all, you will have that calm and warm contagious glow. This is the silent way to influence people.*

# Chapter 6

# Stretch Marks: The New Mother's Worry

Marilyn, a favorite and long-standing patient of mine, was eagerly anticipating the birth of her first child. She came into my office in her seventh month of pregnancy concerned about bluish marks stretching across her abdomen. She asked, "Dr. Buchbinder, what can I do to avoid these stretch marks?" Unfortunately, there is not much my patients can do to prevent and avoid the stretch marks associated with pregnancy. But I explained to her how it is they are formed.

Stretch marks, otherwise known as striae, may appear as pink, bright red, or bluish slightly raised or welt-like marks. Later on they may look flat and smooth or turn into wrinkly white lines. The common areas affected are the outer aspect of the thighs, buttocks, breasts, outer aspect of the upper arms, and abdomen.

Stretch marks commonly occur at puberty, during pregnancy, and following excessive weight gain. There also seems to be a genetic and hormonal susceptibility to striae formation.

Stretch marks result from thinning of the uppermost layer of the skin (the epidermis) and destruction of the collagen and elastic fibers of the lower layer of the skin (the dermis).

## THE COCOA BUTTER CONTROVERSY

The myth that cocoa butter will prevent stretch marks has persisted for generations. Many women also swear by vitamin E, and I have even heard of women who rub expensive designer-label AHA creams on their stomachs during pregnancy.

My own feelings and experiences on this myth is that moisturizers always help reduce the appearance of fine lines. I recommend twice a day moisturizer treatments. However, while cocoa butter might reduce the appearance of stretch marks, it will not prevent them or "cure" them.

But what about women who applied cocoa butter throughout their pregnancies and afterwards had perfectly smooth skin? My opinion is this points to genetics. If you examine the physiology of stretch marks, an external cream could not truly prevent them. But these women may, in fact, be genetically predisposed to not getting stretch marks. Therefore the cocoa butter has been a placebo of sorts. Also, they may have had a pregnancy in which they gained 30 pounds, whereas another woman might go through her pregnancy and gain 45 to 50 pounds.

But, my personal philosophy points to the inner self. Pregnancy can be a wonderful and beautiful time in a woman's life. She may project a glow and inner happiness that transcends anything so tangible as stretch marks. Enjoy your pregnancy! When you hold your baby at the end of those nine months, you'll forget all about stretch marks.

Stretch marks may disappear or become less conspicuous over time. However, in certain cases, they may become a persistent cosmetic problem.

There is no known cure for stretch marks. Sudden increase in size of body parts is a common underlying factor in the case of pregnancy, puberty, and excessive weight gain. I am not aware of any surgical procedure done today to correct stretch marks. However, there are surgical procedures available to remove excess skin. Short of surgery, I recommend regular moisturizing of the skin to lessen the wrinkly appearance of stretch marks (refer to section on Dry Skin). The use of aloe vera or cocoa butter does not prevent stretch marks but they serve the purpose of moisturizing the skin.

**⁊⁊**

## Ligaya On . . . Time

*Do you ever feel sometimes that you are pushing an unmovable wall? You have done everything right but you are just not getting there? Sit tight. This may be the time to do nothing. Let Nature take its course. There is the right time for everything.*

# Chapter 7

# Eczema: Soothing Your Rash

I rene came into my office complaining of a horrible itching and a red rash that worsened whenever she applied make-up, perfume, or hairspray. After talking and examining the rash, I learned that Irene was in the process of looking for a new job. Stress was aggravating a condition I diagnosed as eczema. As always with my patients, education was important. I explained to Irene just what eczema is, and then we devised a treatment plan to bring her relief from this troublesome condition.

Eczema is a common skin condition characterized by rough, red, oozy skin. The condition usually itches. It may involve the hands, feet, legs, arms, trunk, face, or the scalp. Certain cases of eczema may start at infancy. Eczema may occur on and off all through an individual's life. Or in certain cases, an individual may outgrow eczema.

Exposure to skin irritants such as chemicals, skin allergens, and perfumes may provoke an outbreak or exacerbation of eczema. Stress, also, may make eczema worse. Generally, there are two types of eczema — the allergic type and the irritant type. The allergic type

*&*

## Ligaya On . . . Loving Yourself

*One of the most important lessons that I learned is to love myself.*
*It is very difficult to genuinely project love to another human being*
*without a true love for oneself. It is natural to share a cup that is*
*running over. Helpful step: Look at your face straight in the mirror*
*every morning and tell yourself out loud "I love you." Repeat three*
*times. Face the day . . . beautiful inside and out.*

is either an immediate type or the delayed type (refer to chapter on
Dry Skin). The irritant type usually occurs within minutes or a few
hours.

A good example of an immediate type of allergic skin reaction is
when someone's lips or throat suddenly swells up after eating something or taking a pill that this particular person is allergic to. An
example of a delayed type of skin allergic reaction would be if
someone using the same hair dye for a year all of a sudden developed
a rash on the scalp after using the same chemical to color the hair.
An example of an irritant type of skin reaction is a rash that a person
develops immediately after using a certain concentration of glycolic
acid. This person may not develop the same rash if a much lower
concentration of glycolic acid is used. (You can substitute many other
chemicals, creams, etc. Glycolic acid is just one example.)

The rash caused by an allergic reaction may look very much like
the rash caused by an irritant reaction. Many times, I as the dermatologist have to rely on the history and precise description of how the
rash started. In situations wherein the cause of the allergic reaction
is difficult to pinpoint, I use patch testing to more clearly identify the
substance or substances that the person is allergic to.

An allergic reaction may be due to things or substances we touch,
smoke, fumes or mists that we inhale or that settle on the surface of
the skin, and food, drinks or pills that we ingest. It may occur as a
direct allergic reaction due to the substance or it may occur as a
photosensitive reaction which means that sunlight or ultraviolet light
is an added factor in the reaction with the substance producing the
allergic reaction. Irritant reactions are usually due to direct contact
with the substance.

## Possible Causes of Eczema

| Possible Irritants | Products/Chemicals |
|---|---|
| alkalis | soaps, detergents, toilet bowl cleaners, lye, ammonia preparations |
| acids | vinegar, phenol, salicylic acid, L-ascorbic acid, trichloroacetic acid, alpha hydroxy acids (AHAs), tannic acid |
| metal salts | |
| chlorine | |
| fluorine | |
| cutting oils | |
| petroleum derivatives | |
| tar | |

### Possible Allergens

| | |
|---|---|
| poison ivy, oak, sumac | |
| lanolin | wool fat, wool wax, cosmetics |
| neomycin sulfate | Neosporin®, commonly found in triple-antibiotic creams or ointments |
| epoxy resin | may be found in adhesives, product finishing, laminates |
| plants | mango, philodendron, primrose, chrysanthemum |
| nickel sulfate | earrings, bracelets, rings, coins, nickel-containing alloys |
| chromates | shoe leather, gloves, zippers, paint, cement, musk ambrette |
| ethylenediamine | Aminophylline®, hydroxyzine, tripelennamine, piperazine antihistamines |
| bismarck brown | dyeing silks, wools, leathers |
| formaldehyde | nail polish, textile finish, paper, disinfectant, insecticides |
| turpentine oil | furniture polish, cleaning fluid, paint thinner |
| mercurials | mercurochrome, in some weed killers, insecticides, preservatives in eyewashes, nasal jellies, suppositories, amalgams, thimerosal |
| mercaptobenzothiazole | rubber accelerator |
| products of bacteria, fungi and parasites | |

### Possible Causes of Cosmetic Dermatitis

| | |
|---|---|
| antiperspirants | aluminum chloride, chlorhydroxide, zinc salts, quarternary ammonium compounds, zirconium preparations |

## Possible Causes of Eczema *(continued)*

| Possible Irritants | Products/Chemicals |
|---|---|

**Possible Causes of Cosmetic Dermatitis**

| | |
|---|---|
| hair dyes | paraphenylenediamine, acid violet, ammonium |
| cobalt | blue tattoo pigment, hair dyes |
| chromium | dyes |
| lead | dyes |
| hair bleaches | peroxides, ammonia |
| hair sprays | lanolin, shellac, gum arabic |
| depilatories | calciumthioglycate, sulfides, sulfhydrates, mercaptans, waxes, resins |
| hair tonics and lotions | tincture of cinchona, tincture of cantharidin, salicyclic acid, resorcin, quinine sulfate, perfume |
| nail lacquers | sulfonamides, formaldehyde |
| artificial nails | acrylic monomers, glue |
| lipsticks | tetrabromofluorescein, allantoin compounds |
| eye make-up | base wax, perfume |
| sunscreen | para-aminobenzoic acid, digalloyl trioleate |
| skin bleach | hydroquinone, kojic acid, alpha hydroxy acids (acts as an exfoliant) |
| mouthwashes | essential oils |
| perfumes | almond oil, coriander, geraniol, heliotropine, hydroxycitronella, jasmine, linalool, lavender, lemon, lemongrass, neroli, origanum, oil of cloves, perppermint, spearmint, wintergreen, cinnamic alcohol, musk ambrette |

The table of possible causes of eczema, or other probable lists for other categories presented in this book, may seem extensive and may give you a feeling that everything you are likely to touch may cause a skin problem. Word of assurance: You will not have a problem with these products unless you are particularly sensitive to specific components of these products. I am providing these lists to hopefully enable you to objectively identify the particular cause of your problem if you happen to be one of those people who have encountered a problem.

Eczema may run in families with a history of eczema, hay fever, asthma, or "sensitive" skin. It is not contagious. However, a secondary bacterial infection may easily occur in eczema especially when

---

### ECZEMA DO'S AND DON'T'S

**Do**

Use a moisturizer daily after shower or bath

Stay away from substances that tend to cause your skin roughness or
rash (refer to Possible Causes of Eczema table)

Consider having a patch test done by your dermatologist or physician
if your eczema is recurrent or persistent

Cut your nails to avoid deep scratches

**Don't**

Leave sores or fissures unattended

Scratch

---

there are cracks on the skin surface. In this case, the bacterial infection may be contagious.

Common treatments for eczema include the use of gentle soaps
such as glycerin-containing soaps without lanolin and regular use of
moisturizers especially after baths, showers, or hand washings. Some
of my recommended moisturizers are Moisturel® Lotion, Eucerin®
Cream, Aquaphor® ointment, Vaseline Intensive Care®, DML Lo-
tion®, and Lachydrin® Five Lotion. The dermatologist, usually, will
recommend the avoidance of allergens or irritants to the skin, and
may prescribe cortisone creams or ointments and antibiotic creams
or pills.

# Chapter 8

# Itching: Relief for Scratchy Skin

I cannot stand itching. I know I am not alone. Universally, itching is probably one of the most uncomfortable sensations an individual can experience. Both itching and pain are mediated by the same type of nerve fibers. A milder stimulus to the nerve produces the sensation of itch and a stronger stimulus produces the sensation of pain.

Why do we scratch when we itch? It is because we want to get rid of that most annoying sensation of itch. By scratching, we substitute a stronger stimulus to that nerve and end the itching by inflicting pain instead. The deeper we dig into the skin, the stronger the stimulus, and the better we feel. What a mess!

Dermatologists are quite relieved when they are able to pinpoint the particular cause of the patient's itching — like an insect bite, a mite, or an itchy rash that can be treated. Many an itchy situation is

&

### Ligaya On . . . The Mind/Body Connection

*Itching tears the skin out. Pain tears the heart out. The mind plays its tricks.*

so annoying and complex that it not only drives the patient crazy but also the dermatologist. There is nothing more challenging to the dermatologist than an itchy patient without an apparent rash.

The most common bug bites that I see in my office are caused by mosquitoes, ants, fleas, and "no seeums." The skin reaction that causes the patient a lot of discomfort is usually due to a sensitivity reaction to the bug bite. Some individuals are sensitive to certain bug bites more than others. Skin reactions may vary from mild itching which goes away immediately to persistent itching for days, welt-like reactions, swelling of the skin, persistent hard bumps, pimple-like bumps, and clear to pus-filled blisters. Pus-filled blisters are usually mistaken for a bacterial infection but is actually due to the sensitivity or allergic reaction to the bug bite. However, I do recommend a bacterial culture, in this case, to rule out a secondary bacterial infection.

Over-the-counter treatment for bug bites include the use of soothing agents which contain camphor, menthol, phenol (should not be used in infants or pregnant women), and alcohol but I recommend the immediate application of 1% hydrocortisone cream or ointment to treat the sensitivity or allergic reaction. Antihistamines like diphenhydramine (Benadryl®) may also help but you should be aware of the side effects of this drug like getting drowsy or tired. People who have glaucoma should not take this drug without their doctor's approval. Persistent or severe reactions should be brought to the attention of your doctor. Secondary bacterial infection may develop after the bites and this needs to be treated with an antibiotic.

It is important to determine the underlying cause of itching prior to treatment for the simple reason that the incorrect treatment may make the condition worse. For example:

1. Hydrocortisone cream which is helpful for bug bites, eczema, psoriasis, and dandruff may worsen a jock itch caused by fungus or an itchy rash caused by scabies.
2. Lanocaine, a topical anesthetic, may cause a skin allergic reaction on top of the original itching.
3. Neomycin, usually incorporated in triple-antibiotic ointments, is a common cause of skin allergic reaction.

---

## ITCHING DO'S AND DON'T'S

### Do

Try the following remedies for soothing:
  plain moisturizers, moisturizers containing camphor (0.3% to 0.5%)
    and menthol (0.3% to 0.5%)
  witch hazel
  cool oatmeal baths
  Sulzberger's household bath oil — 2 teaspoons of olive oil and one
    large glass of milk to the tepid water in the bathtub

### Don't

Shower more than once a day — this can dry the skin
Overdo with too many at-home remedies — you can complicate the
  situation for a dermatologist or physician later on
Scratch
Drive or operate machinery while taking antihistamines that cause
  drowsiness
Use salves containing lanocaine or any of the "-caine" mixtures

---

  4. Calamine lotion, a drying agent, may intensify the itch-
     ing of dry skin.

It is definitely more productive and cost effective to first pinpoint
the cause of the itch prior to medicating. Within this book, I discuss
specific skin problems that may cause itching. Within these chapters,
I have recommended specific over-the-counter remedies for specific
itchy skin problems. I suggest that you approach your search for the
possible cause and treatment in this manner. I wrote this chapter to
point out very common pitfalls and hopefully guide you towards a
clear, efficacious, and cost-effective direction.
     Common soothing remedies are plain moisturizers or moisturiz-
ers containing camphor (0.3% to 0.5%) and menthol (0.3% to 0.5%),
witch hazel, cool oatmeal baths, Sulzberger's household bath oil
which is made up by adding 2 teaspoons of olive oil and one large
glass of milk to the tepid water in the bathtub. Bathing or showering
should be limited to at most once a day and skin should be lubricated

after each shower or bath. Over-the-counter antihistamines such as chlorpheniramine or diphenhydramine may be tried to relieve itching. I recommend taking the first dose at bedtime because most antihistamines can cause drowsiness. Do not take these antihistamines if you will be driving or operating machinery.

Almost every itchy patient who comes to my office usually has tried every home and over-the-counter remedy available. Many times, I must first eliminate the side effects that these remedies have caused the patient before I can get to the real problem of itching. I usually need to analyze the physical, psychological, and social environment of my affected patient in order to offer relief or cure their itching. Whenever I accomplish this I feel rewarded.

# Chapter 9

# Warts: The Toad Myth

Debbie came into my office suffering from warts on her hand. "There are dozens of over-the-counter remedies, but I don't know which to choose," she said. The warts were very obvious. Therefore she wanted a fast remedy, but one that wouldn't cause discomfort. She also wondered how it was she got the warts.

Contrary to myth and folklore, toads do not cause warts. Instead, warts are caused by the human papilloma virus (HPV). Many strains of HPV have been isolated. Most strains of this virus will not cause real health problems. However, a few strains of HPV have been associated with cervical and skin cancer.

Warts may affect any skin or mucosal surface like the mouth, nose, and genital or rectal areas. Common warts may go away by themselves but they may spread and cause some discomfort, especially if they involve the hands or feet. They can also be contagious to others. Direct touching is the usual way warts are spread.

Warts are quite a challenge to treat, especially if they involve the fingers and feet or if they have been present for a long time. Common wart treatments include salicylic acid, lactic acid, trichloroacetic acid, retinoic acid, podofilox, catharidin, podophyllin, cryosurgery, electrosurgery, and other methods of destruction. Some warts may go away on their own without treatment. Warts may keep coming back

---

### DR. BUCHBINDER'S USEFUL TIPS
### ON WART REMEDIES

Tightly wrap the wart with a waterproof tape.
You may change the tape only when it falls off. The longer it stays, the better.
Your skin will turn white and ugly under the tape. This is temporary.
Be persistent in treating warts (may take several weeks to months).
Warts can be spread. Do not pick your warts.

### COMMON ACTIVE INGREDIENTS
### IN WART REMEDIES:

Salicylic acid
Lactic acid

---

after getting rid of them. I therefore recommend that conservative treatment methods that have the least number of side effects, especially scarring, should be tried first.

Salicylic acid and lactic acid are common ingredients in many of the over-the-counter wart remedies. They come in different concentrations as drops that easily dry upon application, or as medicated tape or plaster. I prefer to use the tape or plaster if they fit practically on the wart location because the occlusion (cutting off from air) helps in the penetration of the medication. If you use the liquid preparation, cover it with a waterproof tape, which you may leave on for a few days at a time. Occlusion of the skin softens the upper skin layer, thus making it easier to wash off or wipe off the dead tissue fragments resulting from wart treatment. I have even gotten rid of warts by mere occlusion alone, done over a period of several weeks to several months. If you see my son walking around with a tape around his finger for weeks, we may be trying to get rid of a wart! Just make sure you use a hypoallergenic and waterproof tape. Do not panic if you see your skin turn all white and ugly after removing the tape. This is a natural reaction after occlusion to get rid of dead tissue within the wart in order for the repeated treatment applications to be more effective. Persistence is the secret to efficacy in treating warts. Most dermatologists will tell their patients that wart treatment is usually a long and arduous process, no matter what method we use.

There are certain people who believe hiding a dish cloth will make warts disappear. We can chuckle at this or the toad myth. Not true! See your physician or dermatologist for treatment if the over-the-counter wart remedies have not been effective.

# Chapter 10

# Herpes Simplex I: Treating Your Canker Sores

When I told a patient of mine, Carla, that she was suffering from Herpes simplex I, she seemed embarrassed. "Herpes? How can that be?" "Relax," I told her, "let me explain."

Herpes simplex is a viral infection that can affect the skin or mucous membranes of the mouth or the genitalia. There are two types of Herpes simplex virus — the type I and type II viruses. The type I virus is usually associated with the infections in or near the mouth area while the type II virus is usually associated with infections at or near the genital area.

Type I Herpes virus infections are more common and are most often seen near the mouth area. They are generally referred to as canker sores or fever blisters. This type can affect any age group from children to adults.

Herpes simplex virus infections may be precipitated by sun exposure or periods of decreased body resistance. They may be associated with pain or discomfort. They can be contagious and may be recur-

---

### FEVER BLISTER DO'S AND DON'T'S

**Do**

Apply a lip balm containing SPF 15 or higher prior to sun exposure
   and reapply it every half hour
Rest
Apply ice if the numbing helps soothe the pain

**Don't**

Touch the area
Kiss anyone — you can spread the HSV
Go out in the sun without extra sun protection
Ignore a canker sore or fever blister that lasts longer than two weeks
   — see a doctor

---

rent. Herpes virus may be spread through kissing or directly touching the active sore. A person having the sore on one spot may spread the sore to another spot by directly touching or rubbing. An outbreak usually lasts for a couple of weeks.

There are now available treatments and prophylaxis for Herpes simplex virus infection, such as acyclovir (Zovirax®), famciclovir (Famvir®), and valacyclovir hydrochloride (Valtrex®). Some of these treatments may soon be available over-the-counter. Treatment is either in the form of a pill, a liquid taken by mouth, or a salve. Treatment by mouth is usually more effective. Early treatment of an episode of Herpes simplex also increases effectiveness.

There are two routes of treating Herpes simplex. One form is treating the episode of a new or recurrent breakout. Another form is prophylactic treatment for frequently repeated episodes of Herpes simplex. This latter form usually requires daily treatment for a six-month period. However, neither episodic or prophylactic treatment guarantees that the person will be cured of Herpes simplex (meaning that the person will never break out with Herpes simplex again).

L-lysine, an amino acid available at health food stores in pill form, had been rumored to help in the past. However, from my experience in clinical practice, I do not see a remarkable improvement of the lesions with this remedy.

It is important that you have an accurate diagnosis of Herpes simplex prior to treatment. There is a rapid method of diagnosing Herpes simplex in the physician's office. However, a culture of the virus is necessary to distinguish between Herpes simplex type I and type II. Over-the-counter remedies short of the treatments that I mentioned above are generally not helpful. In fact, I recommend that you not touch the lesions directly in order to prevent spread of the lesions on yourself or to other people. The use of a sunscreen prior to sun exposure can be helpful in preventing a breakout. You may use a lip balm containing an SPF 15 or higher. A water resistant sunscreen lotion or gel may be used instead of a lip balm. I suggest that you wear a hat or carry an umbrella if you tend to have recurrent episodes of Herpes simplex.

# Chapter 11

# Chickenpox:
# The Itchy Virus

I f you had chickenpox as a child, it is likely that you remember the episode very clearly. You were miserable, itchy, ran a fever. In fact, the horrible itching is probably what you remember most. Your mother may have tried numerous home remedies to help you. And everyone admonished "Don't scratch!!"

Chickenpox is a virus infection which can infect children or adults. The incubation period is about 2 to 3 weeks. The rash is often preceded by 2 to 3 days of slight fever, tiredness, headache, sore throat, loss of appetite and dry cough. It usually starts as faint red blotches which become red bumps. These progress to "teardrop" blisters within 24 hours. Successive fresh crops of blisters appear for a few days mainly on the body then on the face or even in the mouth. Initially, the breakouts may be limited to sun-exposed areas. Crusts fall off in 1 to 3 weeks. The rash may be itchy especially in the blister stage.

Chickenpox rash usually should not leave a scar unless it has been scratched or secondarily infected by bacteria.

Chickenpox is contagious. You may also get the chickenpox from someone who has the shingles. Chickenpox is usually more severe

---

### CHICKENPOX DO'S AND DON'T'S

**Do**

Keep your child with the chickenpox home to avoid spread to other
    people
Ask your pediatrician about the chickenpox vaccine
See your pediatrician immediately after the appearance of symptoms
    and signs if you desire effective treatment for the chickenpox
Cut your or your child's nails to avoid secondary infection and scars
See your obstetrician immediately if you never had the chickenpox
    and you are exposed to chickenpox during the first four months of
    your pregnancy
Try tepid baths with 1/4 cup of baking soda

**Don't**

Take aspirin to relieve your symptoms
Scratch

---

when it affects adults. Complications are rare in children but may be
more common in untreated adults.

Maternal infection with the chickenpox virus during the first four
months of pregnancy may result in abnormalities of the fetus. See
your obstetrician immediately if you never had the chickenpox as a
child and you are exposed to the chickenpox during the first four
months of pregnancy. Do not wait for symptoms to appear!

Oatmeal baths, calamine lotion, cool compresses, and antihistamines like diphenhydramine may help control the intense itching.
Tepid baths with baking soda (1/4 cup per tub of water) may also
relieve the itching. Fingernails should be kept short and clean to
minimize injury from scratching and to lower the possibility of a
secondary bacterial infection. Aspirin should be avoided because it
may lead to other disease complications.

Treatment is now available for chickenpox and is most effective
when used early at the onset of the rash. The best news is this disease
may be prevented by a chickenpox vaccine which is now available
and is administered by pediatricians or family physicians.

# Chapter 12

# Shingles:
# The Painful Rash

M aryanne, a 50-year-old librarian, came to my office in incredible pain with a rash of blisters on her left side. She complained of severe itching along with the pain and hadn't been able to sleep the night before her office visit. After discussing her medical history, I asked Maryanne if she had ever suffered from the chickenpox. "As a child," was her reply, "maybe I was 7 when I had them." My diagnosis for Maryanne? Shingles. I carefully explained the cause and appearance of shingles and then prescribed medication for the pain as well as the comforting news that once the shingles went away, she would probably never get them again.

Shingles is a breakout caused by the chickenpox virus. As a rule, you must have had chickenpox prior to breaking out with the shingles. For example, you may have had the chickenpox at age 9 and then develop the shingles at age 45. The shingles is due to the reactivation of an inactive virus that remains within the body long after the outbreak of the chickenpox.

The rash of the shingles usually is seen as a group of blisters located in a line only affecting one side of the body without crossing

---

### SHINGLES DO'S AND DON'T'S

**Do**

Severe one-sided pain + appearance of rash along the painful area
  most likely is shingles — see your doctor immediately

**Don't**

Confuse shingles (Herpes zoster) with Herpes simplex — same first
  name, different disease
Use lanocaine or other "caine" containing salves to ease the pain
Go near children or pregnant women who never had the chickenpox

---

the middle. It may be preceded by pain prior to the rash. The pain
is usually located along the same side where the rash appears later on.

The rash of the shingles usually goes away after a few weeks. The
most dreaded part of this illness is the accompanying pain which can
last for a long time after the rash has disappeared. Pain is due to the
involvement of the peripheral nerves in this disease. The pain may
not occur at all but on the other hand it can be quite intense and
disturbing. Painkillers may or may not help in relieving the pain that
may occur. Pain, on the other hand, may abate or go away on its
own. The duration of pain is very difficult to predict. As a doctor, I
try to help my patients' comfort as much as possible.

A person with the shingles may not spread the shingles to another
person but may cause chickenpox in another person who never had
the disease. Shingles usually occurs only once in a lifetime with very
few exceptions. Shingles may come about for no apparent reason,
although it is not uncommon for shingles to occur after injury to a

ta.

Ligaya On . . . Your Inner Voice

*When you are stuck in a situation with no one to turn to, do not
panic. Take a deep breath, concentrate on your breathing, and listen
to the silence in your mind. You probably hear or know from your
core what needs to be done. Trust yourself. You are the captain of
your ship.*

particular body part (like the shoulder or hip) or during periods of emotional stress.

Fortunately, prescription medications are now available (acyclovir, famciclovir, and valacyclovir hydrochloride) for shingles. When used properly and started early at the outbreak of the rash, they can prevent a bad outbreak of the rash and lower the possible occurrence of the most excruciating pain that may occur with or follow the rash. Early treatment also renders the patient less contagious (will not spread the chickenpox virus) in a shorter amount of time.

# Chapter 13

# Skin Discoloration: Seeking Smoother Skin

Every person is born with a certain basic skin color. This color is usually enhanced as the person matures. Since our skin is the organ directly exposed to our environment, environmental factors may affect the skin directly or indirectly.

Our skin color is determined by the size, type, color, and distribution of melanosomes in which melanin is produced and deposited. This substance is produced by the pigment-making cells on our skin. The most important factor in the environment that affects skin color is the amount of ultraviolet light exposure to the skin surface. It stimulates the pigment cells to produce melanin. Melanin is difficult to dissolve.

Abnormalities in melanin production or abnormalities in melanin-producing cells bring about abnormalities in skin color. These abnormalities may be patchy or may affect the entire skin. Skin color change may manifest either as a lightening or darkening of the skin. Some of the common skin color changes that are bothersome are freckles or liver spots, melasma (commonly referred to as "mask of pregnancy"), vitiligo (loss of skin pigment), tinea versicolor (white spots due to a superficial fungus infection), and eczema (refer to chapter on Eczema).

**Freckles.**    Freckles (lentigines) or liver spots are one of the most common forms of skin discoloration. It is not uncommon for a patient to walk in complaining about these brown to black spots. The sun stimulates our pigment cells to produce melanin which determines our skin color. Let me make a simple analogy to demonstrate how freckles form: In a patch of gardenias, some are bushier and bear more flowers than the rest despite similar growing conditions. Same with our pigment cells — some cells produce more pigment than others. Some cells get so stimulated that they grow a remarkable array of projections within the upper layer of the skin and are seen as liver spots or freckles. Some are wider and darker than others.

Freckles may get darker with excessive sun exposure. Avoidance of the sun or proper sun protection may lighten existing freckles. Prominent liver spots may be lightened by cryosurgery (lightly freezing with liquid nitrogen) which can be performed by a dermatologist. A superficial chemical peel (refer to section on skin peels) may also lighten or remove the freckles or liver spots.

Another myth I can expose for you: Lemon juice or peroxide will not bleach liver spots. Fading creams are also quite ineffective in fading liver spots. You stand a better chance of lightening your liver spots with regular use of an effective sunscreen than by using a fading cream.

**Melasma.**    Melasma is darkening of the skin in sun-exposed areas. It may occur for no known reason, or it may be associated with pregnancy or in some individuals who are taking birth control pills. The "mask of pregnancy" may disappear on its own without treatment after pregnancy or it may persist. Other associated factors are hormonal dysfunction, cosmetics, and genetic factors. The usual areas of involvement are the forehead, cheeks, temples, and upper lip. Fading creams containing hydroquinone used in conjunction with a sunscreen may be effective in lightening melasma. The use of a sunscreen on top of the fading cream is extremely important because sunlight is definitely a factor in this type of skin darkening.

ta.

## Ligaya On . . . Personal Style

*I came home from an all-night call while I was a surgical intern (prior to my dermatology residency) and found the new sewing machine that I had ordered from a catalog. I was planning to cook for my friends that weekend. I ran out to the fabric store to pick out material for a dress. I had never used a sewing machine on my own nor had I learned to make a dress. But I persevered and I looked great with my hand-made purple dress at the dinner party! I love clothes and I love colors. Aside from camouflage make-up to cover up uneven skin color, you can utilize clothes style and color to enhance your appearance.*

I recommend the use of a sunscreen that blocks both UVA and UVB (discussed in detail in Questions and Answers). Hydroquinone comes in higher concentrations and they are available with a prescription. Hydroquinone may be combined with kojic and/or glycolic acid in skin-lightening preparations. Be careful of skin irritancy in any of the above combinations.

**Vitiligo.**   Color loss in vitiligo may be partial or total. A person with vitiligo is more susceptible to sunburn because of the loss of skin pigment. An episode of sunburn may cause the vitiligo or loss of skin color to spread on the areas that were burned. Skin color in vitiligo may or may not come back on its own. It is extremely important for individuals with vitiligo to stay out of the sun as much as possible or wear a sunscreen that blocks both UVA and UVB.

**Tinea versicolor.**   This usually appears as white spots on the skin of the chest, shoulders, upper back, face or upper arms. Sometimes it may appear as pink or brown spots. It is caused by a superficial fungus (different from the fungus causing "jock itch"). This infection is prevalent in warm areas and the tropics. This fungus has to be differentiated from eczema, vitiligo, and another common condition known as idiopathic guttate hypomelanosis. The latter condition is usually seen as smooth white spots usually occurring on the legs and arms. There is no known cure for this latter condition.

56                                          Skin Care: Clear & Simple

## Dr. Ligaya Buchbinder's Skin Discoloration Guidelines

| Skin Condition | OTC Treatment | Prescription Treatment | Prevention |
|---|---|---|---|
| Melasma | Hydroquinone in formulation | 4%–8% hydroquinone formulation | Sunscreen, other forms of birth control aside from the pill |
| Vitiligo | None available | Consult your physician | Extreme sun protection, camouflage make-up |
| Tinea versicolor | Clotrimazole twice a day | 2 ½% selenium sulfide suspension | Regular use of OTC soap/ shampoo after Nizoral® cure to prevent recurrence |
| | Tolnaftate twice a day | Ketoconzaole (Nizoral® shampoo, cream or pills) | |
| | Salicylic acid with or without sulphur soap daily | | |
| | Selenium sulfide shampoo | | |
| Birth marks & moles | None | Consult your doctor when there is a change in color, size, shape and/or bleeding | Sun protection |

Tinea versicolor responds readily to simple treatment. However, treatment needs to be persistent and thorough to effect a cure. There is a likelihood of recurrence due to incomplete eradication of the fungus. Over-the-counter antifungal creams or liquids that are quite effective in getting rid of the fungus are clotrimazole and tolnaftate. I recommend twice-daily applications covering the entire affected area for at least a period of two weeks. I also recommend the use of 3% salicylic acid with 3% sulphur soap (Stiefel® — available over the counter) for the entire body for a period of one to two months and periodically thereafter to help prevent recurrence of the rash. It is wise to shampoo the hair regularly with selenium sulfide shampoo to eradicate the fungus from the scalp where it usually resides without necessarily causing any scalp trouble. Selenium sulfide 2.5% suspension is also effective when applied to the affected areas and left to dry overnight and washed off in the shower the morning after. Care should be taken not to apply this in the genital area and other delicate areas such as the groin, face, and underarms. This treatment sometimes may irritate the skin and if this happens, immediately rinse it off and apply a soothing moisturizer.

**Birth marks and moles.**    Almost all of us have birth marks or moles somewhere on our bodies. They are other forms of discoloration on the skin. Birth marks and moles may be flat or raised. These spots will not disappear with the use of salves. Removal of these growths usually requires some form of surgery. There are very few birthmarks or growths that disappear on their own.

*Word of caution:* If any blood relative has a history of malignant melanoma and you have some moles yourself, it is a good idea to at least have them looked at by your physician. Even if you do not have a family history of malignant melanoma but you notice a change in color, size, shape, or bleeding in an existing or a new growth, mole, or birth mark, I suggest that you have it looked at by your physician.

Consult your physician regarding skin color changes not responding to your own remedies. This is a situation wherein a trained expert is valuable in diagnosing and treating your particular problem. A good word of advice in color-changing situations is try to avoid the sun. Protect yourself from it before you even see a physician.

# Chapter 14

# Skin Cancer: The Danger in the Sun

$\mathcal{S}$uzanne, a 40-year-old blue-eyed and blonde executive, came to see me to ask for advice on skin care. She was unhappy about the "crow's feet" at the corners of her eyes, the deep wrinkles on her upper lip, and the rough texture of her skin. "How come my skin is never smooth?" As soon as I took a look at her skin, I knew that she was a victim of the sun. "But I love the sun — why can't I expose my skin to it?" I looked closer at her entire skin surface, especially the sun-exposed parts and I found a pearly papule, tucked in the crease on the left side of her nose. I saw some fine blood vessels through this translucent growth. I asked Suzanne if or when she noticed this growth. "Oh, that is a bump that I thought was a pimple but it has been there for over a year." I suggested to her that I should do a skin biopsy because this growth had several characteristics that made me highly suspect a skin cancer. She agreed to this and sure enough, it was a form of skin cancer — a basal cell carcinoma. We took care of this problem and, fortunately, I made the diagnosis soon enough before the skin cancer really had a chance to grow larger and deeper.

≈

### Ligaya On . . . The Sun

*My husband and I travel to the Orient twice a year. We both have a deep affinity for the Orient so that it almost feels like we have lived there in many lifetimes together. My brother made a joke before our wedding that he thought Charles must have been an Oriental prince in one of his past lives. We are fortunate enough to be able to purchase a very small island off the mainland where I was born. This place was never inhabited and is surrounded by a magnificent coral reef. Natural Bonsai trees grow within the rock formations on the island and my brother and his wife did a phenomenal job in preserving its natural beauty and ecology. This place exudes so much "magical" energy that just getting there makes you feel that you have landed on another dimension. This is one place on this planet that you can watch the sunrise and the sunset while sitting on the same spot! As you can see, I am the "daughter" of the sun — but I do cover up with sunscreen so I don't get burned.*

Just like many things, too much of something you love may be detrimental to you. One important factor that concerns us all is the occurrence of skin cancer. Scientific research has repeatedly shown that ultraviolet rays can induce skin cancer formation. It also has shown that ultraviolet rays' effects on the skin is cumulative. This means that the amount of sun damage that we have when we are 50 is the accumulation of the excessive sun exposure that we received since we were born. It also has been shown that a bad sunburn may lead to skin cancer many years down the line. If our mothers only knew then, they would not have left us in the stroller unprotected from the sun for too long.

Each individual skin has a certain threshold for total ultraviolet ray exposure. If this threshold is surpassed, skin cancer may develop.

". . . but can you just tell me how much sun I can take?" Unfortunately, I do not know that magic formula, nor does anyone else.

What should we do then? Take the sun with caution and use a lot of common sense. Just remember how the prune looks while you arc on your beach blanket on the scorching sand! And if that sand is scorching, just think what the sun is doing to your skin!

I, too, love the outdoors. I love to be out on a clear day playing tennis, water-skiing, or windsurfing. We can still enjoy these pastimes. Our children can still grow up enjoying the outdoors. There is one difference — now we know better. Now, we can protect ourselves from the sun with any or a combination of the following:

1. Use a good sunscreen with at least an SPF 15. When you are going to sweat a lot, use a sunscreen labeled water resistant. Note that SPF 15 means that the sunscreen offers 15 times longer sun protection to the skin compared to not using any sunscreen at all. Reapply the sunscreen after a couple of hours, especially if you are in and out of the water or if you are perspiring. Remember, there is no complete sunblock except a physical sunscreen like titanium dioxide or zinc oxide. There is no sunscreen that completely protects you all day without reapplication.
2. Wear a hat or use an umbrella to offer added protection. Make sure your ears are protected.
3. Wear protective clothing.
4. Avoid direct sun exposure during the middle hours of the day (between 11 A.M. and 2 P.M.).
5. An increased resistance of the unprotected skin to solar radiation can be achieved by slowly increasing your time of exposure. This means that on your first day on the beach during your tropical vacation, do not exceed 10 to 15 minutes of direct sun exposure without other forms of sun protection. You may stay out approximately 40% longer the next day until a maximum of one hour exposure time has been reached. Skin types I and II (see table) run the risk of burning despite this precaution.

Certain individuals can take more sun before burning compared to others. The skin type classifications in the table will give you an idea of how you may compare with the rest of the population. This

## Skin Type Classification[a]

Skin Type I — Always burn, never tan
Skin Type II — Usually burn, tan less than average (with difficulty)
Skin Type III — Sometimes mild burn, tan about average
Skin Type IV — Rarely burn, tan more than average (with ease)
Skin Type V — Brown-skinned, rarely burn, tan easily and profusely
Skin Type VI — Dark-skinned, generally never burn, tan profusely

[a] Adapted from Reference 14.

classification is based on redness and tanning to first exposure in mid-day sun for 3/4 to 1 hour in northern latitudes in the summer.

# Chapter 15

# Psoriasis: Help for Distressed Skin

Jack came in to my office complaining of flaky, itchy skin on his hands, as well as a stiffening in the knuckle joints of his hands. He had delayed seeking treatment, thinking at first it was a reaction to new detergent. His condition progressively worsened however and the itchy condition was also on his scalp — something he originally thought was dandruff. I spent some time with Jack, asking questions about his family medical history. While questioning Jack, he remembered that his grandmother had also suffered for years from a similar itchy condition. Jack and I reached the same conclusion. He was suffering from psoriasis.

Psoriasis is a disorder in skin proliferation meaning the amount of time it takes for the bottom layer of the skin to shed on the surface. It is characterized by the build-up of scales and redness underneath the scales.

Normally, it takes 2 to 3 weeks for the bottom layer of skin cells to shed to the surface. In psoriasis, it only takes 2 to 3 days. Because of the faster than normal turnover of the skin cells from the bottom layer, a thickening and build-up of scales occurs.

## DR. BUCHBINDER'S RECOMMENDED
## PSORIASIS REMEDIES

Tar solution/soap/bath/shampoo (refer to end paragraph in Dan-
    druff chapter for tips on how to use tar on your scalp)
Sunlight
The application of oil (i.e., mineral/olive/vegetable/coconut) to the
    skin improves the diffraction of sunlight as it hits the skin, thus
    making the light treatment (with or without tar) more efficacious
Avoid a sunburn!
1% hydrocortisone cream/ointment/solution applied at least 2–3
    times daily
Salt water/bath loosens the thick scales (dissolve a pound of salt in the
    bathwater)
Salicylic acid soap/shampoo
Take a break or a fun vacation in the sun when you are under a lot
    of stress
Think positively — worry can make your psoriasis worse

Psoriasis is usually an itchy condition but it may occur without
itching. It may flare up at times of stress. It can affect the skin
anywhere from the feet up to the scalp. Scratching the skin may make
psoriasis worse. This disorder can also affect the nails. It may even
attack the joints, causing arthritis. Psoriasis is not contagious, but it
may run in some families.

Common treatments for psoriasis include tar, ultraviolet light,
anthralin, cortisone, and derivatives of vitamins D and A. Current
medical researchers are looking into the treatment of psoriasis by
manipulating the patient's immune system. The positive effects of
alpha and gamma interferons have been linked with psoriasis.

Ultraviolet light or sunlight is the most common and most an-
cient treatment for psoriasis. Studies on the effects of ultraviolet light
on the turnover of skin cells have repeatedly shown that ultraviolet
light slows down the rate of skin cell turnover. In other words,
sunlight slows down the shedding of cells from the bottom layer to the
surface of the skin. This beneficial effect of the sun on skin cell
shedding prevents the thickening and build-up of scales in psoriasis.

Unfortunately, the effects of sunlight on the skin is a two-edged sword. On one hand it helps psoriasis, while on the other hand it can damage the skin and eventually cause skin cancer (refer to chapter on Skin Cancer). This is a dilemma for me as a dermatologist. There are a multitude of other treatment options which are utilized for psoriasis. Ultraviolet light certainly should not be excluded but it should be utilized with caution and proper monitoring. As a practical person, I certainly believe that many beneficial things in life when consumed or utilized in excess may become detrimental.

Tar either in the form of wood tar or coal tar is an old-fashioned remedy for psoriasis. These tars contain a great variety of compounds, most of which are not well-defined. Tar in combination with sunlight enhances the ultraviolet B effect on the skin, thus increasing the susceptibility of the skin to the positive effects of ultraviolet B (UVB) in the case of psoriasis.

*Word of caution:* Due to this enhancing effect of tar on UVB, a bad sunburn is likely to occur if tar is used without extreme caution. From my own personal observation, the use of tar alone improves psoriasis even without direct sun exposure after application. Tar is available in the form of an oilated bath, bar soap, or a gel that is directly applied to the skin. Treatment should be done on a daily basis. Try the cheapest tar preparation first. In bathing, use a capful of an oilated tar bath in a tub of water and soak in it for 15 to 30 minutes. Try not to rinse your skin after the bath — just pat your skin dry because the small amount of tar absorbed on your skin will continue to give you its beneficial effects the rest of the day. Using a bar of soap containing tar in the shower gives you a similar effect. Apply a moisturizer on your skin, preferably containing some kind of oil like mineral oil when you get out of the shower. And now . . . a Dr. Buchbinder cost-saving tip: You may even use straight mineral oil, olive oil, or vegetable oil! If you go out in the sun, you have to remember that you may burn more easily than usual because of the tar left on your skin. The oil on your skin will improve the light diffraction as it hits your skin, thereby improving the efficiency of the light treatment in combination with tar. The direct sun exposure of psoriasis-involved skin is beneficial for psoriasis. Just be careful not to get a sunburn. Protect the rest of the skin that is clear of psoriasis with a sunscreen, especially

your face. You may apply other salves like hydrocortisone after you
dry your skin.

Dissolving a pound of salt in the tepid bathwater helps in thinning the thick build-up of scales. You may also soak in the ocean for
a natural salt bath. A vacation on a remote tropical beach is one of
the best getaways for anyone suffering with psoriasis! Isn't that a
wonderful doctor's perscription? At the beach, if you are lucky enough
to live in or be able to travel to a warm climate, you can bring your
tar gel, tar shampoo (refer to the last paragraph in the Dandruff
chapter), tar bath oil, or tar soap bar with some oil to rub on your skin
prior to sitting every day on the beach (make sure you apply the tar
gel after soaking in the ocean). There, you just designed yourself a
real enjoyable modified psoriasis regimen! In the old but still reliable
Goeckerman regimen for psoriasis, the dermatologist puts you in the
hospital, covers your entire body with crude coal tar 24 hours a day
and puts you in a light box while slowly increasing your length of light
exposure daily. This is usually a 21-day regimen, or maybe shorter
depending on your response.

*Word of caution:* The combination of tar and sunlight is quite potent.
Be sure to ask your physician or dermatologist for specific guidelines
prior to undergoing this modified regimen yourself in order to avoid a
severe case of sunburn, enough to ruin your entire vacation and
enough to cause skin damage and skin cancer later on in life.

Hydrocortisone (.05% to 1%) is available as cream or ointment
over-the-counter. I prefer the 1% ointment preparation for psoriasis.
Hydrocortisone is the least potent of all the cortisone preparations
available short of a prescription. I advise a two or three times a day
application for psoriasis, regularly done over a period of at least three
weeks, unless the rash disappears prior to three weeks.

Psoriasis can be temporarily cured or put into remission with
proper treatment. There are many other alternatives in the treatment
of psoriasis aside from the readily available things that I have discussed. In general, I would like to comment that most of these
treatments range from fair to good. Psoriasis is a chronic illness and
may range from localized to widespread. Some patients are able to
deal with this illness very well, however, some patients are plagued

and overwhelmed with this malady. Many patients who have walked into my office ask me a straightforward question in the form of a statement as they walk into the door — "I came here to find out whether there is anything new for psoriasis. I have tried everything available under the sun and I still have my psoriasis." My gut reaction to such a statement is a feeling of awe. I wish that science could give me all the answers but my pocket is empty many times when confronted with such difficult questions. If there is an effective prescription for every illness, maybe we do not need a doctor but a computer printer. As a doctor, I feel that I should function as the healer. If I cannot heal the physical illness, maybe I can try a key to unlock the portal of the heart.

There is one important factor quite important in psoriasis that I would like to mention. As a dermatologist, I find that one of the most common factors that is associated with a flare-up or persistence of psoriasis is emotional stress which may or may not be recognized by the patient. It is not uncommon for a patient to tell me that there is really nothing bothering them beyond the ordinary. What is ordinary to one may be extraordinary to another. Does our body and mind (both conscious and subconscious) have its own separate standard for ordinary? How about an integration of the body, conscious mind, and subconscious mind? In my own personal preference of terms, I refer to this as the integration of the body, mind, and spirit. Maybe the portal of this integration is through the heart. If all else fails, this is certainly an avenue worth looking into. Science may lack the explanation for this integration since we are dealing with "relatives" and the "imaginary." Maybe you can come up with at least a personal testimonial of disease improvement with personal inner work.

ža

### Ligaya On . . . Change

*It is good to change your routine once in a while. Change paves the way to progress. I love change. Many times I change for the sake of change. Change creates movement, and movement releases energy. Energy leads to transformation. Fresh water constantly flows. Stagnant water leads to disease.*

# Chapter 16

# Fungus Infection: Stomping Out Athlete's Foot and Jock Itch

I live in the paradise of Boca Raton, Florida. We have steamy summers and mild, warm winters. Compared to colleagues in other areas of the country, I see a tremendous number of patients with fungal infections because fungi thrive in warm, humid conditions on the skin. And nowhere will you find it steamier than South Florida in August! People who work out naturally sweat more here, and even those of us standing still find it very hot and humid.

Athlete's foot and jock itch are commonly caused by a skin fungus. There are several types of skin fungus but, in general, they respond to a common treatment. As I said the fungus loves to thrive under warm, moist conditions on the skin. This infection may be itchy. Most patients come in with complaints of persistent dryness or scaling on the feet or groin that are not relieved with regular applications of a moisturizer.

Fungus is generally contagious although some individuals are more susceptible to fungal infections than others. The tendency for

---

# FUNGUS INFECTION DO'S AND DON'T'S

## Do

Dry your feet, groin, and other body creases well after shower or bath
Dry skin using a hair dryer set on moderate
Try clotrimazole cream twice a day to entire affected areas
Try applying undecylenic acid powder to your feet and footwear on a
  daily basis
Try to wear new footwear after your athlete's foot is cured
Consult your physician regarding a cure for persistent fungus

## Don't

Use salves containing hydrocortisone on affected areas
Walk barefoot in bathrooms, showers, or even on floors and carpets

---

skin fungus may even run in families. Fungus is usually spread by
fungal spores which thrive in warm and moist areas. Fungal spores
can be physically destroyed using extremely high burning tempera-
tures. This means that if your athlete's foot is cured, you may get it
back by wearing your old contaminated shoes!

There are several over-the-counter fungus treatments available
like clotrimazole, undecylenic acid, miconazole, tolnaftate, and nystatin. Prescription antifungal creams and oral medications recommended by a dermatologist or physician generally eliminate the
fungus more efficiently. I usually recommend the use of clotrimazole
cream twice daily for a period of two to three weeks.

Word of caution: The use of salves containing hydrocortisone
may make your fungus worse! After the fungus clears, I recommend
the use of medicated powder containing undecylenic acid or
miconazole after thoroughly drying the affected area with a cotton
towel.

Remember: fungi love to multiply in warm and moist areas. The
occurrence of fungal problem usually increases in the summertime.
I recommend the use of flip-flops when taking showers in public
places. Fungal spores are quite difficult to eradicate short of extremely high burning temperature. Therefore, it is quite difficult to
eliminate fungal contamination. Certain people are prone to contact

fungus infection. This tendency may even run in families. Proper drying of the skin after bath or shower is important. The use of medicated powder (i.e., undecylenic acid powder) on the feet or groin for the fungus-prone helps lower the occurrence of reinfection.

Try to eliminate contaminated footwear after your fungus is cured. Make sure to check with your dermatologist prior to getting rid of your contaminated footwear because what may seem to be cured for the layman may not be cured in the eyes of the expert. There are tests available to the dermatologist or physician to objectively determine cure in addition the clinical eye. Numerous salves and pills are available with a prescription to cure persistent fungal infections.

# Chapter 17

# Yeast Infections: Dispelling the Yogurt Myth

Carol came to my office complaining of a moist, white rash in the corners of her mouth. After talking, she disclosed that she had recently finished a two-week course of antibiotics to treat a throat infection. Upon examining her rash close up, I discovered the culprit. Carol had a yeast infection.

Yeast infections of the skin are commonly caused by the yeast Candida albicans. This organism thrives in warm and moist areas of the skin surface. The summertime usually brings a rush of patients to the dermatologist's office with infections involving the groin, under the breasts, folds under the abdomen, and the underarms. Other common yeast-infected areas are the vagina, in between fingers or toes, tongue, and inside and corners of the mouth. The infected surface usually looks red or white, slightly scaly, moist and may have scattered pimples which may appear pus-filled. The areas affected may be itchy.

Oral Candidiasis or "thrush" may occur in newborns or adults. The inside of the mouth and the tongue may be involved. The tongue may look smooth, glazed, and bright red. The specific case of thrush in an infant needs the attention of your pediatrician. In adults, the infection frequently extends to the corners of the mouth to form "perleche." Perleche commonly occurs with ill-fitting dentures due to drooling at the corners of the mouth especially while sleeping. You may treat localized Candida at the corners of the mouth with clotrimazole cream applied after breakfast and at bedtime. The physician usually treats extensive oral Candidiasis without difficulty.

Diaper rash due to Candida usually starts around the anus and spreads over the entire area. The irritation is enhanced by wet diapers. For an infant with diaper rash, I recommend frequent and timely changing of wet diapers. The rubbing of petrolatum around the anus after wiping may help the irritation and as the irritation abates you may apply clotrimazole cream twice a day. You may apply the petrolatum on top of the clotrimazole cream. I do not recommend the use of talcum powder to this area or any area in infants due to the danger of them inhaling the talcum powder which can be hazardous to their health.

Another cause of yeast infections is prolonged intake of antibiotics. Unfortunately, if this is the cause, there may not be much you can do to prevent it because if antibiotics are necessary for another condition, then you just have to bear with this side effect.

Once you contract a yeast infection, the most common remedy includes keeping the affected areas dry and open to the air or separated with an absorbent material like cotton cloth. Using a hair dryer with moderate temperature setting after showers or bath may help. Medicated powders containing nystatin or undecylenic acid are helpful in preventing infections under the breasts, groin, or between the toes. Over-the-counter medications like clotrimazole, miconazole, tolnaftate, nystatin, and gentian violet are helpful in eliminating the infection, when used properly. I recommend a twice-daily application, following the directions on the label.

Eating yogurt does not prevent yeast infections of the skin. This old wives' tale has persisted for some time. The yeast infection is topical. Treating it by ingesting a food will not help it go away.

---

## YEAST INFECTION DO'S AND DON'T'S

### Do

Dry the creases on your body thoroughly
Eat a balanced diet
Change wet diapers immediately
Try clotrimazole cream twice a day to externally affected areas
Avoid constant soaking of hands in water
Stay in a cool place during warm weather
Inform your physician if you are prone to yeast infections
Seek a pediatrician's care in cases of thrush in infants

### Don't

Use talcum powder with infants
Use hydrocortisone without proper guidance from your physician.

---

Malnourishment may be a cause of recurrent yeast infections aside from an underlying predisposing factor like diabetes, debilitation, or immune deficiency. In the case of persistent or recurrent infections, it is best to seek the help of your physician.

# Chapter 18

# Common Vascular Anomalies: Dealing with "Spider Marks," Red Blebs, and Stork Bites

## Spider Marks

Spider marks, medically known as spider telangiectasias, are spider-like webs of prominent small blood vessels (small arterioles) with a red dot in the center. This is sometimes referred to as "broken capillaries." These are not the same as the "spider veins" that are part of varicose veins seen on the legs.

Spider marks may appear as a single spot or in several spots and are usually seen on the face, neck, and chest. They may occur in normal skin and even in children. They may also develop in areas of injury. Spider marks may appear during pregnancy.

Lesions in healthy children may persist indefinitely but a small proportion disappear by themselves. Lesions that appear during pregnancy may disappear 6 weeks after delivery but can reappear in subsequent pregnancies. The appearance of numerous spider telangiectasias may be associated with liver disease.

Estrogen hormone plays a role in the development of some telangiectasias. In my experience, I see this problem more frequently among women.

Treatment of spider marks may be done in the physician's or dermatologist's office with some success. Some cases may recur more than once after treatment. Treatment utilizing a fine needle and low intensity electric current is a simple method that is often used. This treatment directly eliminates the central small arteriole and its finer branches in an instant! (The process is called electrodessication.)

## Cherry Angiomas

Shari, a 30-year old hairdresser, came to my office because red marks seem to be popping out on her body. Upon looking closely, I counted about 30 small, circular ruby red lesions ranging from the size of a pin head to the size of a water droplet. These were located on her trunk, thighs, arms and one presented itself right on her forehead. I made the diagnosis of cherry angiomas. I reassured Shari that the majority of 30 year olds (both male and female) most likely will find one of these on their skin. They are not dangerous and they do not turn into skin cancer. This is the most common vascular anomaly and the occurrence increases with age. Cherry angiomas are easily obliterated with light electrodessication or freezing with liquid nitrogen. She decided to have me treat the cherry angioma on her forehead because it really bothered her. She felt reassured about the rest of her lesions and she decided to leave them alone.

## Port-wine Stain (Nevus flammeus)

The most common type of port-wine stain is what we refer to as Nevus flammeus nuchae or "stork bite." This occurs in over 5% of the population and is usually located on the back side of the upper portion of the neck and is usually partially covered by the scalp hair. This stain usually appears as a red patch of skin which may or may not blanch completely upon applying direct pressure on the skin surface. We usually leave this type of port-wine stain alone.

Midline nevus flammeus or "salmon patch" is located on the middle of the forehead at the frown line or on one upper eyelid. This is common in infants. This form tends to fade or disappear during childhood.

Port-wine stains occurring on the trigeminal nerve distribution (the 5th cranial nerve) of the face are usually larger and are quite uncommon. Although the surface of this port-wine stain is smooth, small bumpy or warty outgrowths may be present or develop in the course of life. This type of port-wine stain may be hereditary and may be associated with other abnormalities in the eye and/or the brain. I highly recommend that you consult a physician regarding this type of port-wine stain. Port-wine stains may now be improved by laser surgery. The argon laser is usually used for this condition.

ঽ৯

## Ligaya On . . . Nature

*Sometimes I wonder why human skin color does not change like a chameleon's. Is it because we are capable of changing clothes and wearing different hairstyles and make-up? Or is it because Nature knows that the color of our skin does not matter. Nature is certainly quite liberal and wise!*

# Chapter 19

# Impetigo: Beware the Contagious Infection

J ason, a 7 year old, was brought in by his mother because of fast-spreading blisters. "I don't think it can be chicken pox," she said. "He had them a year ago." Most of the blisters I examined on Jason were located on his face, neck, and hands. Upon close examination, these blisters were discrete and thin. Most of them had ruptured and were covered by golden yellow crusts. Some of the crusted lesions look like cigarette burns. Some blisters contained pus. I immediately suspected a case of impetigo. I took a skin culture and sure enough it grew *Staphylococcus aureus* bacteria.

Impetigo is a skin infection commonly caused by the *Staphylococcus* bacteria. *Streptococcus* bacteria may also cause impetigo. Impetigo is a highly contagious skin infection and is quite common. It may affect children as well as adults. It is usually seen as small blisters or it may look like cigarette burns. Swelling of the lymph nodes is common in Streptococcal impetigo. Group A beta-hemolytic streptococcal skin infections are sometimes followed by an acute kidney involvement. This occurs in about 2% to 5% of the early childhood cases (usually before the age of six).

## IMPETIGO DO'S AND DON'T'S

### Do

Keep your pets clean
Cut your child's fingernails regularly
Teach your children when and how to wash their hands properly
   from an early age
Wash contaminated towels, clothes, and linens separately
Sterilize beauty salon implements
Properly chlorinate swimming pools
Treat yourself if you are an asymptomatic carrier of *Staphylococcus
   aureus* bacteria
Consult a physician immediately when you suspect impetigo

### Don't

Touch a blister with bare hands
Expose the infected child to other children until proper diagnosis and
   treatment is made
Share towels

Common sources of infection for children are dirty fingernails, pets, and other children they are directly in contact with. Adults may get it from contaminated barber shops, beauty parlors, public baths, swimming pools, and infected children.

Proper diagnosis and treatment by a physician is extremely important in order to prevent the spread of this disease and prevent other complications. There are some individuals who may not have active impetigo but are carriers of this bacteria especially in their nostrils. These individuals need treatment in order to prevent spread of the *Staphylococcus* infection to direct physical contacts. The use of antibiotic ointment (for example, Bactroban® ointment, Polysporin® ointment) in the nostrils of a carrier is highly recommended. It is important to obtain a bacterial culture in a spreading infection to determine the specific oral antibiotic which is effective in eradicating the bacteria. Short of a culture, the physician usually uses a broad spectrum antibiotic to eliminate the bacteria.

Disinfecting with povidone iodine solution or hydrogen peroxide 3% and applying an antibiotic ointment containing polymyxin B (for example, Polysporin® ointment) twice daily with a Q-tip to a localized lesion may control a mild infection. (This routine is also effective in taking care of common cuts). However, impetigo is a fast-spreading infection and is highly contagious. If the rash is starting to spread, it is wise to immediately seek help from your physician. Avoid sharing towels or bed linens with a person who has impetigo to minimize the possibility of spread. Contaminated towels, clothes, and bed sheets should be washed separately with soap and hot water.

# Part II _____
# The Hair: Our Crowning Glory

# Chapter 20

# Introduction: Our Crowning Glory

Our scalp hair is our crowning glory but hair may not necessarily be an asset someplace else on our body.

Hair at different body parts grows at different rates. Scalp hair, for example, grows at a rate of about 1/2 inch each month while thigh hair grows at a rate of 1/4 to 1/3 inch each month. Scalp hair grows faster in women than in men, but body hair grows faster in men than women.

Each individual hair grows in three different growth cycles — the resting stage lasting from 3 to 4 weeks (telogen), growing stage lasting on the average of 3 years but may range from 2 to 6 years (anagen), and the transitional stage between growing and resting lasting about 1 to 2 weeks (catagen). Each hair has a genetically predetermined lifespan as well as maximum potential length. This means that your strand of hair is eventually shed anywhere from between two to six years.

Under normal conditions, hair that is shed is replaced by new growth. A person may normally shed anywhere from 50 to 100 hairs a day. This amount of hair shed is replaced by new growth. Daily hair

ﾞ

## Ligaya On . . . Making Mistakes

*It is OK to make mistakes. A mistake makes a great teacher. I love
to take chances because whatever is the outcome, I always win. I
either attain my conscious goal or I grow from the lesson I learned
from my failure. I urge you to experiment. Try a new hairstyle. Have
a manicure and pick a color that suits your mood. Try a different
color make-up on a night out. Change your look on the next season.
See how it feels. It may be uncomfortable or you may feel self-
conscious at first but keep trying. It feels great to get in the groove!*

loss above this number is considered excessive and is therefore not
normal. However, hair may shed more during certain seasons of the
year like the fall.

Body hair takes a shorter time to complete its cycle as compared
to scalp hair, therefore, body hair does not grow quite as long as scalp
hair.

There are two different types of body hair — the lanugo hair
which is finer and shorter sometimes referred to as "peach fuzz" and
the terminal hair which is coarser and longer. The finer facial hair is
referred to as lanugo hair and the coarser hair like the beard is
referred to as terminal hair.

A number of hormones have been shown to affect hair growth in
various ways from increased hair growth to hair loss (for example,
testosterone, prednisone). A wide variety of medications may bring
about temporary hair loss (for example, colchicine, heparin, coumarins,
vitamin A, propranolol). There are many other medications that may
cause hair loss. Word of advice: If you are taking a new medication
and you notice an increased amount of hair loss, bring it to the
attention of your physician.

Contrary to popular belief, neither shaving nor menstruation has
any effect upon hair growth rate.[2] Shaving does not make the hair
grow thicker or faster (refer to chapter on Hair Care). Therefore, a
woman who shaves excess hair on her chin will not grow a man's
beard.

Graying of hair is due to the decrease in the amount of pigment
on the strand of hair. Pigment cells are absent in the root of white

hairs. By now you know I like to dispel myths: Plucking a grey hair does not cause two to grow in its place. Premature graying may run in families or may be associated with certain autoimmune diseases such as pernicious anemia or thyroiditis. It may also occur in vitiligo (refer to chapter on Skin Discoloration). Normal graying of hair occurs with aging. The age of onset of normal graying is genetically defined and may be different in general age of onset with different races. There are well-documented reports claiming extremely rapid ("overnight") graying of hair. From my own personal observations, I do believe that stress may cause premature graying of hair.

# Chapter 21

# Common Hair Problems: Too Little Hair or Too Much

## Hair Loss

Hair loss occurs when the rate of shedding is faster than the rate of regrowth. In other words, when you lose more than 100 hairs a day over a period of time you may develop baldness or you will have thinning of the hair. This hair thinning may be temporary or permanent. A person usually does not perceive real thinning of the hair until 50% of the hair has been lost.

If you are concerned about losing too much hair, I recommend a daily hair count of the hairs dropping off the scalp in order to know whether or not you are truly losing too much hair. You may do this by counting the hairs on your shower drain, brush, pillows, etc.

Hair loss is classified as either temporary or permanent. Permanent hair loss usually is due to damage, malformation, or destruction of the hair follicles so that they can no longer produce hair.

The following sections will discuss the common types of hair loss.

### *Male-pattern or Female-pattern Baldness*

My father was bald at an early age — so was my uncle. My brother who is now 48 years old has very thin hair on his crown and his frontal hairline has receded considerably. The worst part of this genetics deal is that it is also affecting me! My hair is generally about half as thick as it used to be. The best way for me to tell is when I tie my hair up in a pony tail. Do you have one of those circular rings to measure the amount of spaghetti to cook? I used to measure for two portions and now my hair measures for one portion.

Male- and female-pattern baldness are the most common forms of hair loss. Male-pattern baldness manifests a little differently from female-pattern baldness. Both often occur with a family history of hair loss in either sex. Therefore, if a woman's father has baldness, this woman may have the tendency for female-pattern baldness.

Hair may recede on the front hairline and may start thinning on the top of the scalp. As these two areas continue to lose hair, the person may end up with baldness on the front and top of the scalp or crown. This usually happens among men. Women usually lose hair by general thinning in these areas and it is quite uncommon to see a definite bald spot among women. Instead, we see the sparsity of hair in these areas and we see the scalp through a thin head of hair in women.

Medication (Rogaine®) is available for this condition but the results usually are not as much complete regrowth as we like it to be. Consult your dermatologist or physician regarding this treatment, now available over the counter.

Another alternative is hair transplant. Hair from your scalp is harvested from the back portion which is genetically not destined to be lost and transplanted on the front and the top of the scalp where hair is permanently lost. Ask your surgeon regarding this procedure as well as its side effects. Another alternative is to wear a wig or hairpiece. There are several methods now available to attach a wig or hairpiece successfully. A hair professional can help you achieve a natural look with these methods.

### *Patchy Hair Loss: Alopecia Areata*

Michael, an active 7-year-old boy, was brought in by his mother to see me with a round bald spot on the crown of his head, the size of a dollar coin. His mother practically saw his hair fall off in a clump. She was petrified when she saw this and she ran to her pediatrician right away. She was prescribed a salve for fungus which she diligently applied twice a day. This did not help and she was afraid that Michael would infect his younger sister with this fungus. I looked at the bald spot, examined the rest of Michael's skin especially all the hair-bearing areas like the arms, legs, and eyebrows. This was the only spot where hair was missing. I scraped the surface of the bald spot to examine the scrapings under the microscope for fungus. The examination was negative for elements that will suggest a fungal infection. Besides, the bald spot was nice and smooth with some of what we call exclamatory pointed hair. This specific hair abnormality is seen in alopecia areata.[3] I prescribed mometasone furoate lotion for Michael to be applied daily. I saw him back in two months and some terminal hairs were starting to grow out of the bald spot. I saw him back in six months and the bald spot was completely filled in with short terminal hairs. A year later, Michael and his mother were smiling as they walked into my office because his hair had grown and you could never tell that he used to have a bald spot. He came in this time for me to treat his wart. As we parents know . . . it's always something!

Alopecia areata is characterized by sudden hair loss in clumps resulting in single or multiple bald patches. In severe cases, hair loss can be total which means loss of the entire body hair. Partial hair loss may affect any hair-bearing area of the body like the scalp, eyebrows, eyelashes, beard, moustache, pubic hair, underarms, or general body hair. Sometimes the hair loss can be quite rapid becoming widespread within a number of days.

Both sexes are equally affected and alopecia areata may occur at any age.

When a small number of bald patches are present, there is a better chance of the hair growing back. This may happen within six months to a year. Reoccurrence of hair loss may occur.

A number of modalities are available which have resulted in hair regrowth. Cortisone preparations in the form of liquid or creams are often utilized. Hydrocortisone 1% liquid or cream available over-the-counter applied twice a day may be tried.

### Telogen Effluvium

This is another condition that causes temporary hair loss following certain stressful events like high fever, blood loss or shock, childbirth, discontinuation of birth control pills, crash dieting, and severe emotional stress. Unlike alopecia areata, there is no treatment. Hair may regrow within 6 to 12 months.

### Dietary Deficiency

A deficiency in protein is another cause of diffuse hair loss. The remaining hair is brittle, dull, and easily shed. Iron deficiency, zinc deficiency, essential fatty acid deficiency and certain digestive absorption problems may also bring about diffuse hair loss.

Word of caution: For those of you who are on a strict vegetarian diet, make sure that vegetable protein and essential fatty acids derived from beans, nuts and other sources as well as vitamin and mineral supplements are included in your diet.

### Other Common Causes of Hair Loss or Hair Breakage

"I went to the beauty salon an hour ago to have my curls relaxed. I went in with a full head of long hair and I walked out with short hair without getting a haircut." You have just experienced hair breakage due to a chemical. Chemicals can alter the bonds that link our hair molecules together and cause hair breakage instantaneously. This is quite a dramatic and upsetting reaction but the good news is your hair most likely will grow back just the way it was over a period of time. Hair usually grows about 1/3 to 1/2 of an inch each month.

Heat is another possible cause of hair breakage. Common sense will tell you that excessive heat can ruin your hair or turn it to smoke altogether! Persistent use of hot combs may not only damage your hair shaft but it may cause deeper injury to the hair root due to heat penetration, thus, causing permanent hair loss in affected areas.

Temporary hair loss has been attributed to certain drugs and environmental chemical exposure. Common drugs and chemicals which may cause this are: large doses of vitamin A, heparin, colchicine, boric acid, propranolol, chloroprene, bismuth compounds, levodopa, and mercurials. Hair loss is usually diffuse, and hair usually grows back after avoiding the definite cause.

Pulling or stretching of the hair may cause patchy hair loss or broken hairs. Common causes include tight pony tails resulting in thinning of the front hairline, hair weaving, rollers, hair clips, or tight braids. Traction alopecia or hair loss due to pulling is usually reversible in the early stages, but if prolonged may result in permanent hair loss.

## Excessive Hair Growth

Tonya came into my office to seek treatment for a rash on her arm. As she was checking out of the office, she noticed the Ligaya® Eyebrow Revolution display on the counter. She was so fascinated by this product because for the first time, she saw a miniature razor designed to remove unwanted facial hair, especially designed for women. She was unhappy with her bushy eyebrows and prominent dark hairs on her upper lip area — another aspect of appearance favored in other parts of the world perhaps, but not thought of as attractive in the United States. She was so thankful to find a safe, easy and painless product that she can use as an alternative to tweezing or waxing. Of course she asked the question of whether shaving will make her hair grow faster or coarser. I reassured her that contrary to popular belief, shaving does not make hair grow faster or coarser (refer to chapter on Hair Care).

Excessive hair growth is noted in women when the pattern is more typical of that seen in men. The boundary between normal and abnormal hair growth is not precise since there is a wide racial and ethnic variation in hairgrowth. Facial, abdominal, and thigh hair are common among Middle Eastern, Southern European, and Russian women, and therefore is considered normal within this background.

If you are experiencing this problem, consult your physician because there may be an underlying cause to your hairiness which can be corrected. Underlying causes of excessive hairiness may include ovarian, pituitary, and adrenal malfunction or tumors.

For individuals who are uncomfortable with hairiness, there are a few options available. For hairiness on the face, you may bleach these hairs as long as bleaching does not cause any irritant or allergic reaction to your skin. Since shaving does not make a woman grow a man's beard (refer to chapters on Hair Care and The Hair), you may shave excess hair. You may also try waxing, but I do not recommend waxing on the facial area because of the dangers of burning and eventual scarring with hot wax. Tweezing, waxing, or close shaving may cause ingrown hair (refer to chapter on Ingrown Hair).

# Chapter 22

# Dandruff: Soothe Your Scalp, End Your Flakes

Lisette is a popular model in Miami. She has long, dark hair. She also has dandruff. Lisette came to me when a big assignment was going to take her on the road for several weeks. "I want to make sure I can manage this condition because I just can't have flaking when the camera focuses on my hair!" she bemoaned. Upon examination, Lisette's scalp was covered with dry and greasy scales distributed in small to larger pinkish yellow patches. The patches were thickest at the back side of her scalp, but patches were also found scattered over the rest of her scalp. She also had some scaling on the crease of her nose and inside her ears. I made the diagnosis of seborrheic dermatitis. I assured her that with understanding and careful attention, her dandruff would be controllable.

Dandruff (seborrheic dermatitis) is another disorder of skin proliferation. Like psoriasis, there is also an increased speed of cell turnover in dandruff. As a consequence, in dandruff cases, we see a build-up of oily scales over reddened or pink skin.

This condition may affect the scalp, back of the ears, the external ear canal, the face, the hairy area of the chest or in rare occasions it may affect the entire skin. It is usually itchy, especially when affecting the scalp. Like psoriasis, dandruff is a chronic problem. This means that the treatments available may control dandruff but the condition usually persists indefinitely. Scratching your scalp may make dandruff worse.

Dandruff may affect infants, children, and adults. Dandruff in an infant is termed the "cradle cap." The appearance may vary from mild yellow or brown scaling to a thick greasy, dirty crust sometimes with an unpleasant odor. I recommend applying mineral oil or a salt solution with gauze or a thin washcloth to soak the thick crusts prior to washing with a baby shampoo. The thick cradle cap usually goes away as the infant matures.

As I like dispelling myths, let me end another one: Dandruff is not contagious.

Now let's examine common dandruff treatments. These include shampoos containing tar, selenium sulfide, zinc pyrithion, resorcin, and salicylic acid. Hydrocortisone 1% liquid or cream available over-the-counter applied twice daily helps improve the condition. Severe cases may require a dermatologist's or physician's care. Word of practical advice: If you are suffering from dandruff, wash your hair regularly (daily or every other day). You may use your favorite hair conditioner after shampoo. Regular shampooing with the use of your favorite shampoo may be all you need to minimize the problem to an acceptable level of comfort (refer to section on Hair Care). In more severe cases, try any of the shampoo types (ingredients) that I mentioned. Apply the 1% hydrocortisone liquid twice daily to the affected areas of the scalp. Switching shampoos once in a while may help in cases of flare-ups. Try not to wear dark clothing if you do not want your flakes to show. Comb your hair

---

### COMMON ACTIVE INGREDIENTS IN DANDRUFF SHAMPOOS

Tar
Selenium sulfide
Zinc pyrithion
Salicylic acid
Resorcin

## DANDRUFF DO'S AND DON'T'S

### Do

Wash your hair daily or every other day with the shampoo of your
   choice
Try tar shampoo in more severe cases
Try alternating shampoos to give your hair a break
Try soaking your scalp prior to shampooing with either of the
   following, depending on the severity of your dandruff — salt
   solution, mineral/vegetable oil, or a capful of tar bath oil diluted in
   1/2 cup of tepid water
Try applying 1% hydrocortisone solution twice a day to badly affected
   and/or itchy areas, especially after shampoo
Use a hair conditioner after shampoo

### Don't

Scratch
Wash your hair less than twice per week
Wear dark clothing when you are flaking
Use hot oil treatments

before you put on your clothes if you are flaking. Hot oil treatments are
not necessary for dandruff. If you have thick crusts or scales on your
scalp, similar to what I suggested for cradle cap, you may soak your scalp
with mineral, vegetable, or olive oil or a salt solution which you can
prepare yourself by dissolving 2 to 3 tablespoons of salt in a cup of tepid
water. You may leave it on for 15 to 30 minutes while wearing a shower
cap, then shampoo your hair with a tar shampoo. (See . . . I have given
away another Dr. Buchbinder inexpensive secret!) Another way of using
tar is by diluting a capful of any brand of a tar oilated bath in 1/2 cup
of tepid water and apply it on your scalp by gently but thoroughly
massaging with your fingers, preferably while wearing thin plastic gloves
(just like coloring your hair). Leave it on 1/2 to 1 hour or preferably leave
it on overnight while wearing a shower cap using old pillow cases and bed
sheets just in case you stain them. Shampoo your hair after either with
a tar shampoo or if you are tired of smelling tar, you may use your
favorite shampoo and then condition your hair.

# Chapter 23

# Ingrown Hair: The Close Shave

Roscoe, a basketball star, has everything going for him. He has a full head of curly hair and a handsome face. There is just one thing about his appearance that really bothers him. He is constantly breaking out in bumps on his beard area. He had what we call pseudofolliculitis barbae. His condition improved tremendously when he grew a beard.

Pseudofolliculitis barbae manifests as bumps usually located on the beard area or any other hair-bearing area. It results when hair tips penetrate the skin rather than passing through the pore or hair opening onto the skin surface.

Close shaves, tweezing, or waxing predispose to this condition.

Depilatories may lessen the chance of this occurrence but the most effective treatment is allowing the hairs to grow beyond the skin surface.

Tip on shaving: Shave with the direction of hair growth, not against. Do not aim for a close shave, thus allowing the leading end of the hair to clear the skin surface. Use a good lubricant while shaving in the form of a shaving cream or gel. I prefer the use of a shaving gel because it allows you to see the hairs and skin that you are shaving.

Tweezing or waxing remove hair from its root. Both these methods may also predispose you to ingrown hairs. Trimming the hair with scissors close to the surface is one method of avoiding ingrown hairs.

Ingrown hairs may develop a secondary bacterial infection because surface bacteria easily colonizes and multiplies given favorable conditions for growth. A disrupted hair follicle in the case of an ingrown hair is certainly a favorable place for bacteria to multiply. In this case, you may need to take an antibiotic by mouth if the infection is not controlled by antibacterial applications. Your physician or dermatologist will most likely take a bacterial culture prior to prescribing the appropriate antibiotic, or he or she may decide to start you on a broad-spectrum antibiotic.

ஃ

## Ligaya On . . . Aches and Pains

*I tend to ignore my minor aches and pains because I feel a lot of them will go away with my positive motions. It is like shaking a rug. A lot of dust will come off!*

# Chapter 24

# Lice: The School Pest

Ever since my daughter was in nursery school, nearly every year we receive a school warning that some children in the classroom are infested with head lice. Last year I was informed by the teacher that the school nurse found head lice on my daughter. Knowing all the implications of head lice to my family, I was really upset by this news. As soon as my daughter came home from school, I sat her under a good light and meticulously examined her hair. A sigh of relief: What the nurse thought were nits were flakes of dandruff loosely clinging on the hairshafts. It is certainly a big inconvenience when one member of the family is infested with the head lice because the rest of the members of the household are at risk of getting it. Proper diagnosis is extremely necessary in order to avoid a lot of aggravation. This brought back memories of my childhood when my grandmother painstakingly pulled the nits from my hair and my ouches for each pull.

Lice usually infest hairy areas of the body. The two most common forms are head lice and pubic lice (crabs). Two forms of the life cycle of lice are usually identified on the affected areas. The adult louse is usually seen crawling on the skin surface of the scalp or the pubic area and the nits or eggs are found attached to the hair. Freshly laid nits are located at the bottom portion of the hair closest to the skin and as the hair grows, the nit gets farther from the skin surface.

Therefore, the distance of the nit from the bottom of the scalp hair will give you an idea of how long the infestation has been going on since scalp hair grows at a rate of 1/3 to 1/2 inch per month.

Each variety of louse (head louse, pubic louse, and body louse) has a predilection for certain parts of the skin and rarely migrates to other regions. They attach themselves to the skin or hair and live upon the blood that they suck.

Lice are highly contagious. Do not share combs or brushes to prevent spread of head lice. Educate your children so that they do not share combs or brushes with playmates or schoolmates. Body lice and pubic lice are also easily spread by direct contact or touching contaminated clothes, beddings, or towels.

Common treatments for lice include lindane (Kwell®), permethrin (Nix®), and pyrethrin (RID®). It is important to get rid of the nits either by using a fine-tooth comb or by picking them individually in order to prevent reinfection after treatment. Removal of nits may be made easier by soaking the hair in vinegar, diluted half and half with water. Avoid contact of medication to your eyes. Wash used clothes, beddings, and towels in the hot cycle of your washer or boil them. Dry cleaning may destroy lice on garments. Dry heat is equally effective in killing the lice and their eggs on clothing. Word of caution: Check your garment or linen label for proper washing instruction to avoid ruining them.

# Chapter 25

# Tender Care for Your Hair

A person with trouble-free skin or scalp hair can usually use most of the shampoos and hair conditioners in the market. I examined at least half a dozen shampoos at random and noted down their individual active ingredients aside from the common solvents and preservatives that they used. I found that these shampoos have common ingredients with slight variations in some of the compounds, namely: water, sodium/ammonium lauryl sulfate, lauramide/cocamide DEA, glycol strearate/distearate, cocamidopropyl betaine, hydrolyzed protein/collagen/silk protein, citric acid, sodium chloride/sulfate, and fragrance. Several shampoos added panthenol. I noted the ingredients of at least half a dozen hair conditioners and I noticed a tremendous variation in their ingredients. I bought four of them and tried them on my hair and my hair did feel different after rinsing the variety of hair conditioners. One of them made my hair feel very smooth and heavy (not much bounce). Another made my hair feel smooth, shiny but lighter than the previous conditioner. Another gave excellent body to the hair, especially after blow drying. Another felt very light and thin but

---

## COMMON INGREDIENTS
## IN SHAMPOOS

Water
Sodium/ammonium lauryl sulfate
Lauramide/cocamide DEA
Glycol stearate/distearate
Stearic acid/glycerin
Cocamidopropyl betaine
Vegetable oils/coconut oil
Hydrolyzed protein/collagen/silk protein
Citric acid
Sodium chloride/sulfate
Fragrance

---

it did the job of detangling and giving my hair some volume and bounce.

I came to the conclusion that I can use practically any of these shampoos. In fact I prefer a basic and reasonably priced shampoo. I would rather spend the money on the right hair conditioner that suits my hair and specific hair styling need for that particular day. The choice of the right hair conditioner depends on the following: hair texture, straight or curly hair, hair color (natural or dyed hair), hair thickness, hair length, hair quality (damaged or healthy normal hair), and hair style. Also, it is good to switch your hair conditioner occasionally to give your hair a chance to benefit from other helpful ingredients incorporated in other brands. Besides, we usually change our hairstyle once in a while and most likely you will find a better suited hair conditioner for certain hair styles.

Certain individuals with a tendency to have acne breakouts need to stay away from greasy or occlusive hair preparations. If breakouts are more pronounced on the forehead compared to other areas of the face, hair products used should be closely scrutinized. Try to avoid the facial skin when applying hair spray, hair styling gel, or mousse.

Common scalp conditions like dandruff or itchy scalp usually will benefit from regular use of shampoos containing tar or selenium sulfide. These conditions usually require frequent washing of the hair and scalp. Many times, you may not need medicated shampoos as long as you wash your hair and massage your scalp thoroughly while shampooing daily or every other day. Use a hair conditioner to prevent drying and splitting of the hair. Cut your hair to a manageable length to facilitate washing and drying.

Shampoos and conditioners may range from a few dollars to expensive brands. My rule of thumb with shampoos and conditioners is for you to use what feels good for your hair. I personally refuse to spend more than a few dollars for a 4-ounce bottle of shampoo or hair conditioner. I recommend the use of a hair conditioner because it seals in the moisture in the hair shaft and it makes it easy for you to comb your hair. A trial of several brands is the best way to find out what suits your hair. Remember: There is no shampoo or hair conditioner to date that will make your hair grow more quickly or thicker. Do not waste your money on shampoo or hair conditioner additives that supposedly will make your hair grow faster!

In general, curly, coarse, thick unruly hair may benefit with added fats (stearic acid/glycerin) and/or oils (vegetable oil/coconut oil). These substances tend to weigh hair down, plus they lubricate and add shine to hair.

Hydrolyzed starch and/or protein add volume to hair, therefore benefitting straight or curly, thin, fine, short or long hair.

Emulsifying wax also creates shine and glide in hair, thus benefitting long, straight hair.

---

## FACTORS THAT MAY AFFECT YOUR CHOICE OF THE RIGHT HAIR CONDITIONER

Hair texture
Straight or curly hair
Hair color (natural or dyed hair)
Hair thickness
Hair length
Hair quality (damaged or healthy normal hair)
Hair style

The mark of an excellent hair conditioner for fine, straight, thin, and long hair is made when it is able to create volume, shine, and glide without weighing the hair down.

Thick, coarse, unruly hair benefits from a hair conditioner that creates glide and weight and this is usually achieved by a formulation containing fats and oils.

I personally use Mane 'n Tail Shampoo and Conditioner®. It does a good job with my long, fine, thin, and straight hair. Despite the fact that the conditioner contains coconut oil, glycerin, vegetable oil, emulsifying wax, and lanolin, it does not weigh my hair down. I am sensitive to some lanolin preparations and I have acne but this conditioner does not bother my skin. Lanolin may bother some individuals who are lanolin-sensitive. I try not to let the conditioner drip on my face when I wash it off my hair. This type of conditioner will be suited for most hair types because it is well-balanced. Oils and fats in hair conditioner may aggravate the acne-prone skin. It is also good to switch your hair conditioner once in a while, especially if you find your hair is getting weighed down.

Certain individuals may be allergic to hair preparations like hair dye. The component of hair dye which commonly causes this problem is para-phenylenediamine. It is good practice to have a patch test before using hair dye especially if it contains para-phenylenediamine.

Grooming of body hair is achieved with the use of different modalities like shaving, waxing, the use of chemical depilatories, electrolysis, bleaching, or plucking. Each of these modalities is used as a matter of personal preference, depending on the body area that needs to be groomed.

Shaving does not make hair grow thicker or coarser. Hair, growing in different body areas, is predetermined genetically to grow a certain way in different stages of a person's life. At puberty, body hair like the beard and pubic hair turns coarser and thicker due to the hormonal changes going on at this age. During this time, in certain cultures girls start to shave their legs and boys start to shave their beard and mustache areas. We see the changing hair characteristics at this time which coincides with the practice of shaving. This explains the mistaken belief that shaving makes the hair grow coarser and thicker.

Eyebrows frame the eyes. Eyebrow styles range from pencil thin, arched to thick lines. The traditional methods of tweezing and waxing both pose the risk of permanent damage to the hair because both these methods involve pulling the hair from the root. Therefore, repeated tweezing or waxing to shape the eyebrows may permanently damage the brows. Now, there is an eyebrow shaver specifically designed to fit the contour of the eyebrows. This enables you to shape your eyebrows painlessly without permanent damage to hair. At your convenience, you can alter your eyebrow style with the changing fashion. (For further information on the Eyebrow Revolution/Brow Shaver, call 561-393-1926 or write to Ligaya Corporation, P.O. Box 4171, Boca Raton, FL 33429-4171).

# Part III

## The Nails:
## Putting Our Best
## Hand Forward

# Chapter 26

# The Nails

*Cut your nails on:*
  *Monday for news,*
  *Tuesday for a pair of shoes;*
  *Wednesday for wealth,*
  *Thursday for health;*
  *Friday for woe,*
  *Saturday for a journey to go;*
  *Sunday for evil.*

Nails, which are hard and durable, protect the end of the finger and serve as a multipurpose tool and weapon.

From the cuticle area to the tip, it may take fingernails from 3 to 6 months to grow out completely and toenails from 4 to 12 months to grow out completely. Nails grow slower as we get older. Nails come in different shapes and thicknesses. Seasonal changes and moderate temperature variations do not have much effect on nail growth.

The cuticles serve a protective function to the nail matrix or the growth center of our nails. Therefore, it is not a good idea to cut or lift our cuticles because this can lead to nail infection and disturbance of nail growth.

Studies investigating the use of gelatin to increase the hardness of nails have been unable to substantiate a positive effect. The calcium content of nails is only 0.2% by weight and most of it is found on exposed nail surfaces. Studies have shown that calcium is not responsible for hardness of nails.

## Common Nail Problems

### Nail Splitting

The most common cause of splitting of the nails at the tip is constant soaking and drying of the nails all day. This can be prevented by wearing waterproof gloves while your hands are in water. However, certain individuals may exhibit nail fragility with nails that break off at the free edge for no apparent reason. Wearing a clear coat of polish does not help a split nail. The use of an acrylic coat or glue may help an accidental nail split but this will not stop the problem of permanent nail splitting. A nail split can act as a focus of nail fungus or bacterial infection due to the disruption of the nail bed. Consult a dermatologist or physician if you have a persistent nail split that does not go away despite your remedies and following my suggestions on nail care.

### Ridging of the Nails

This may be seen in old nails, however, this can also be a result of damage to the nails. This deformity is usually permanent.

### Nail Pitting

This is seen as pin-size indentations on the nail surface. It usually occurs in conditions that involve the nail fold area which is near the cuticle. This may occur in eczema, psoriasis, and alopecia areata. If you have persistent nail pitting and you would like to have beautiful looking nails, you may use acrylics or nail polish as long as you realize the way your nails will look temporarily when you remove the acrylic coat (refer to Chapter 27). Prior to application of nail polish, you should use a coat of ridge filler (ask a beauty supply store or your manicurist) in order to have a smooth nail surface prior to application of the nail polish.

### Lifting of the Nail

This may affect the entire nail or part of the nail. The lifted nail may be discolored white, yellow, green, brown, or black.

The more common reason for lifted nail is nail infection either due to fungus, yeast, bacteria, or a combination of these. However, nail lifting may be due to other causes such as an allergic reaction to nail applications (acrylics, nail polish), drug reaction, or tumor growing underneath the nail. A secondary infection usually sets in when the nail is lifted.

Common over-the-counter treatments include the use of clotrimazole, nystatin, and undecylenic acid applied underneath the infected nail. I usually prefer the use of clotrimazole liquid and this is used by applying one or two drops under the lifted nail in the morning and at bedtime. Do not use a toothpick when applying the drops. Let it seep in with the force of gravity. Treatment should be done twice daily over a period of a few months since it takes 4 to 6 months for the fingernails to grow out. Avoid constant soaking of the hands in water. Try to wear waterproof gloves while doing wet housework. Minimize handwashing. If these treatments are not successful in eliminating the problem, consult your physician or dermatologist.

### Nail Thickening

Most cases of nail thickening are due to fungus. There are cases wherein the nail thickening is due to an inherent abnormality of the nail and is untreatable. Nail fungus can be treated. A new generation of drugs against fungus is available. These drugs are quite effective in treating fungus of the fingernails and toenails when taken by mouth. Two of these drugs that work beautifully are Terbinafine HCl (Lamisil®) and Itraconazole (Sporanox®). Of course the older generation of antifungal drugs still work but, according to my experience, not as efficiently as these two drugs. Ask your dermatologist or physician about these new prescription drugs.

### Nail Discoloration

Nail discoloration is a condition usually attributable to a particular cause. Common causes of nail discoloration are the following: constant use of nail polish, smoking, nail infection caused by yeast, bacteria, or fungus, nail injury, intake of certain drugs, and illness.

Nail discoloration due to a mild nail injury, nail polish, smoking, or the intake of certain drugs usually will go away after resolution of the injury, stopping of nail polish, smoking or the drug. Remember: Allow at least 4 to 6 months for the discoloration to go away after stopping the cause because it takes this long for the nail to grow out. In the case of nail infection due to yeast or fungus, I prefer the use of clotrimazole solution (refer to section on Lifting of the Nail) if the discoloration is underneath the nail (this is usually a white or yellow discoloration combined with lifting of the nail) and the use of clotrimazole cream if the discoloration is on the surface of the nail (this is usually a white discoloration on the nail surface). A green discoloration seen underneath the nail is usually due to a secondary bacterial infection called Pseudomonas (usually in combination with lifting of the nail). In this case, you may try soaking the nail in white vinegar for 3 minutes twice a day and apply 1 to 2 drops of clotrimazole solution underneath the nail after soaking (refer to section on Lifting of the Nail). Dry your nails well after washing. You may use a hair dryer or a hand dryer. Consult your dermatologist or physician regarding persistent nail discoloration despite your remedies because most of these cases can be cured.

### Paronychia (Swelling Around the Nail Fold)

This is one of the most common nail problems seen in the dermatologist's office.

This is characterized by swelling, redness, pain, and separation of the nail fold which is the area around the cuticle. It is due to infection from bacteria, yeast, or fungus.

This problem commonly results from injury to the cuticles or the nail fold. The cuticles serve to protect the nail fold, therefore, cutting, pushing, or biting the cuticles easily lead to this problem. An ingrown nail also leads to this problem.

Treatment includes the use of the proper medication for bacteria, yeast, or fungus. In severe cases, the nail fold needs to be opened up and drained to release the build up of pus.

# Chapter 27

# Nail Care: For Ten Perfect Nails

N ail care is usually simple. Clipping of the nails should be done carefully, avoiding injury to the surrounding skin and cuticles. I do not recommend pushing or cutting of your cuticles because cuticles serve as protection to our nail matrix. Pushing or cutting of the cuticles may lead to a very common nail infection we call paronychia (refer to section on Paronychia). Try not to clip deep at the corners of the fingernails. You may round up the fingernail corners with a nail file. Cut your toenails straight in order to avoid ingrown nails. You may file the corners for a slight taper. I do not recommend cutting the cuticles. If the cuticle is rutty, then carefully trim with the proper instrument (nipper or curved nail scissor). Never rip your cuticles because you may wake up with a throbbing pain or swelling around your nail (refer to section on Paronychia).

Nails can be dressed up with nail polish. However, give your nails a chance to recover from nail polish, especially if you notice some surface yellowing of the nail plate (refer to section on Nail Discoloration). Let the nail grow out completely in the case of discoloration due to nail polish. Word of caution: If you develop a rash around the nails or on the upper eyelids, you may be allergic to the nail polish. Formaldehyde is a common preservative in nail polish that may cause the problem. Certain nail polishes do not contain formaldehyde. Check the labels. For those who are not allergic to nail polish components, one polish is just as good as the other. Always check for possible nail lifting (refer to section on Lifting of the Nail).

If you desire fancier looking nails, there are several options now available — silk wraps, acrylics, and artificial "glue-ons." A flat or spoon-shaped nail now can be made to look fit for a TV nail polish commercial. I always envied those women with perfect nails on the nail commercials. Now I know that you too can have those perfect nails. All you need is a good nail technician and skin that is not sensitive to glue! However, if you do these things on a regular basis, be assured you will run into trouble at some point. Trouble may range from lifting of the nail or nail infection to temporarily destroyed nails. Even one application of a full set of acrylic nails will temporarily destroy the surface of your nails upon removal of the acrylic. These nails usually will grow out and return to normal after 3 to 6 months assuming that no nail infection sets in. I advise you to give your nails a break when you use acrylics, nail wraps, or artificial nails because these adhere to your nails like a barnacle and they may just destroy your nails temporarily. Make sure that your nail technician sterilizes his or her instruments to avoid infections. The superstition which says that "sometimes a manicure can lead to bad luck" may just come true if your technician is not careful!

# Part IV

## Ask Dr. Buchbinder:
## Your Skin Care
## Questions

Questions and Answers

# Questions and Answers

**Q:** What is soap?

**A:** Soap is a cleansing agent made from animal and vegetable fats, oils and greases. It is a salt formed when the fatty acid is mixed with an alkali. Oils and fats used are compounds of glycerin and a fatty acid such as stearic or palmitic acid. Tallow used in soap-making ranges from the cheapest grades, recovered from garbage and used for cheaper soaps, to the best grades used for fine toilet soaps.

**Q:** What is the function of soap?

**A:** Soap functions as a cleansing or purifying agent. The use of purifying agents dates back to the Old Testament. Jeremiah 2:22 states . . . "For though thou wash thee with nitre, and take thee much soap, yet thine iniquity, saith the lord God." Soap removes grease and other dirt by acting as a link between water and grease or dirt, thus loosening the grease or dirt from the surface to be cleaned. These substances are otherwise not soluble in water, therefore, without soap, these substances do not wash away from the surface with water alone.

**Q:** How should I clean my face?

**A:** Use a mild, low residue, perfume-free soap and tepid to cool water. Individuals with eczema and rosacea may use soap-free cleansers usually in lotion form (Cetaphil® Cleanser, Aquanil® Lotion, for example). I recommend applying the soap or cleanser on wet skin and rinsing off with water using your hands.

ʔ⅃

## Ligaya On . . . Being Free

*Before I turned 40, I tended to side with the "purists" as far as skin care is concerned. After I turned 40, I tend to be more liberal in my approach to skin care. Why? I realized that life is too short to be stuck in my ways!*

**Q:** Are antibacterial soaps helpful?

**A:** There are bacteria that naturally colonize on the surface of the skin since it is exposed to the environment. No soap or cleanser can render your skin sterile. Nature has provided us with natural resistance to these surface bacteria as long as the skin barrier is not broken.

**Q:** Are moisturizing soaps helpful?

**A:** Moisturizing soaps are fine but they are no substitute for applying a moisturizer to your entire skin when you get out of the shower or bath. I would rather you save your pennies on soap and spend a little extra on a good hypoallergenic, perfume-free, non-comedogenic moisturizer. This seems like a mouthful but manufacturers should place proper labeling on their product to assure appropriate use for the skin-conscious public.

**Q:** What are the most common active ingredients in moisturizers?

**A:** Common ingredients are: AHAs (commonly in the form of lactic acid or glycolic acid), dimethicone, petrolatum (these moisturizers are usually of thicker consistency and tend to be more occlusive), linoleic acid, glycerin, stearic acid, lanolin (I advice sensitive individuals to stay away from this), mineral/ sunflower seed and other plant oils (from my experience, these do not seal in moisture on the skin as efficiently as the first four moisturizers that I have mentioned as an example).

**Q:** How do I keep my skin nice and smooth?

**A:** A disease-free skin simply needs a good moisturizer on a regular basis. Refer above to my choice of a moisturizer. The secret is regular daily use of the moisturizer after showers or baths to seal in the moisture on the skin surface which normally evaporates and leaves the skin dry. Non-soap cleansers (for example, Cetaphil® Cleanser and Aquanil® Lotion) may be used by people who are sensitive to soap (refer to chapters on Acne and Dry Skin). The cost of soap-free cleansers may range from a few dollars to over ten dollars. Check out the cheaper ones first in your local drugstore because the high price tag may not be worth it. Remember, you do not need the added scent unless it is your preference.

Another secret to keeping the skin nice and smooth is the use of a mild exfoliant in the form of a soap or cleanser. Examples are: 2% salicylic acid soap bar (Stiefel®) and AHA washes.

The use of certain skin creams or lotions which cause exfoliation also may help keep your skin nice and smooth. Examples are: vitamin C cream or lotion, AHA cream or lotion, azelaic acid, and tretinoin. You may need a moisturizer while using some of these products, depending on the degree of exfoliation or peeling that ensues. Peeling may range from not visible to obvious. It all depends on the product, its efficacy, and what is suited for your particular skin. Remember: Use a sunscreen when you will be out in the sun.

**Q:** What do you think of a skin peel?

**A:** A skin peel is the systematic wounding of the skin layers using one or more injurious agents (in other words, chemical, laser) This controlled injury to the skin layers prompts regeneration of new tissue and results in skin rejuvenation and partial or complete disappearance of wrinkles, sun damage, and scars. There are three major types of skin peels or wounding.

A preferred classification of agents used in chemical peeling is based on the studies of these agents as used in a variety of techniques.[5] Generally, skin peeling is classified into three types: (1) superficial peel — very light or light, (2) medium peel, and (3) deep peel. Agents used in superficial peeling includes: resorcin, azelaic acid, Jessner's solution (resorcinol, salicylic acid, lactic acid, and ethanol combination), lower concentrations of TCA (trichloroacetic acid), solid carbon dioxide, tretinoin, and alpha hydroxy acids. Agents used in medium peeling include: higher concentrations of TCA alone or in combination with solid carbon dioxide or Jessner's solution, phenol, laser. Agents or methods used in deep peeling include: phenol, laser.

Side effects of the peels vary depending on the type of skin peel utilized as well as your particular skin type. Ask your physician for the possible side effects of the peel and what improvement you should expect temporarily or permanently before deciding which type of peel you should undergo.

A very light superficial peel affects the uppermost surface of the skin which is the top layer of the epidermis. The changes brought about by this method are temporary because a new surface layer grows back from the cells at the basal or bottom layer. Most of the changes on the uppermost surface of the skin are brought about from the bottom layer, therefore, peeling the surface or uppermost layer will usually cause temporary results. Very light superficial skin peels are usually done on a regular basis in order to keep up with the constant turnover of new skin layer arising from the bottom layer. Very light superficial peels do not remove wrinkles (with the possible exception of tretinoin — refer to chapter on Wrinkling and the Aging Skin) because wrinkling is a deep-seated process occurring below the epidermis at the skin layer called the dermis. Very light superficial peels however may minimize clogging of the pores because the peeling process is a result of shedding of the loosened cells that are normally stuck together on the skin layer. During the shedding process, pores may become unclogged. The effectiveness of the unclogging depends on the type and concentration of the specific agent used.

A medium peel is intended to peel off the upper skin layer called the epidermis at about the level of the upper reticular dermis. The basal layer of cells is the important layer from which the rest of the upper skin layers arise. The basal layer is above the reticular dermis. Any destruction or peeling below this basal layer may leave a scar. It also means that any destruction or peeling above this basal layer will most likely provide temporary results because the parent or clone cells at the basal layer remain the same. Superficial skin changes not encoded in these clone cells may disappear permanently. Ask your physician as to which blemishes you should expect to go permanently or temporarily.

A deep skin peel is destruction or peeling to the midreticular dermis. This is the kind of peel utilized to permanently remove some wrinkles or existing precancerous growths on the skin called actinic keratosis.

As I have discussed earlier, wrinkling from sun damage is the result of alteration of the elastic fibers like a rubber band effect. These elastic fibers are located beneath the basal layer of the skin, at the reticular dermis. A deep skin peel, under expert hands removes wrinkles and precancerous skin lesions. However, expect some lightening of your skin color after this kind of peel because as I have discussed in the chapter on Skin Discoloration, pigment cells are located in the basal layer of the skin. By getting rid of the basal layer, we get rid of some of the pigment-producing cells.

If we get rid of our basal layer, where will our skin grow back from after the peel? Some basal layer remains in the hair follicles which are embedded into the deeper layer of the skin. An expert surgeon will make sure that some of these reserves to promote proper healing remain. How brilliant of nature to keep these reserves in case of trauma! Our skin therefore grows back and some skin color returns, but expect a new skin appearance and complexion to occur.

As you can see, medium to deep skin peeling are highly technical and controlled processes and when done under experienced and expert hands can produce wonderful results. Before you undergo this procedure, make sure you check on the proper medical credentials of your surgeon and try to see before and after results preferably in actual patients. Proper medical clearance is recommended prior to this procedure. Like any surgical procedure, you should discuss the risks with your physician before undergoing a superficial, medium, or deep peel and you should have realistic expectations of the possible outcome. A good surgeon will give you definite guidelines on how to take care of your new skin.

**Q:**  What is the best make-up?

**A:**  If you are one of those fortunate people whose skin is not sensitive to make-up ingredients, you probably will be able to wear most of the over-the-counter cosmetics. All you need to do is pick the right color and consistency of make-up that suits your skin. The cheaper products will be just as good as the more expensive products. Try a make-up demonstration by a make-up artist if you want to see how the product will look on your skin before buying it. Make-up counters usually have testers available. Be aware that the colors you see may look differently when applied on your skin. Consistency and ease of application of a particular product are very important. Therefore, product-testing is the best way to find out. If you are to spend your dollars on one or two high-priced items, you better make sure that you buy a product with the right consistency, smoothness without being oily, and the right color for you.

Color foundation may be applied in two ways. One is by using a liquid foundation preferably with an SPF 15 or higher (make sure you are not allergic to the sunscreen in it) and another method is first applying a moisturizer with a sunscreen on your face, let it dry and then apply a tinted or natural face powder either with a sponge or a brush. Make-up artists usually apply the powder foundation with a moist sponge (use a new sponge each time) to achieve an even coverage but you may use a dry brush to dust it over your face if you desire a lighter (may slightly be uneven) appearance. If you like the sun-tanned appearance without actually exposing your face to the sun, you can use a bronzing powder (available in different shades) that may suit your color. You may apply the bronzing powder either directly on the skin after moisturizing, over your foundation, or after the application of pressed powder. Self-tanning lotions are alright to use as long as you are not sensitive to its components. Word of advice: use a tester before buying one and test it exactly where you intend to use it because the resulting color may be slightly different from your own skin.

In recommending combined products like a moisturizer with a sunscreen, I would like to give you a word of caution. You have to be aware of what is combined within a product and you have to be sure that all the ingredients agree with you. A common pitfall in combined products is the inclusion of ingredients that are not suited for you. As an example, the use of triple-antibiotic ointment (containing polymyxin, bacitracin, and neomycin) is a common practice in giving first-aid. If you are sensitive to neomycin, you can end up with a contact dermatitis or eczema. The use of a combination product in this instance is not good practice. I try to recommend good combinations as much as possible to simplify the regimen for my patients because I am basically an empiricist. I rely on my experiences and observations in addition to my stock knowledge prior to giving advice. Can you imagine waking up in the morning and having to apply three to five layers of salves on your face? Myself as a consumer will not do it regularly, therefore, I do not expect my patients to be more compliant than I am. This principle of simplicity is very important to me because when you see a dermatologist, it is not unusual to walk out of the office with a list of instructions and several prescriptions to treat a breakout or a rash. The first question that the patient should ask is what do I apply first and exactly how.

If you are acne-prone, wear water-based, non-comedogenic make-up. Most products will have this on their label. If you have sensitive skin, stay away from perfumed products unless you have used these products over and over without any problems. Pay particular attention to the labels. Preferably choose hypoallergenic products or products allergy-tested on human beings. This will give you a better chance to avoid potential problems. Discard your old make-up after a few months in order to avoid skin infections. When you purchase make-up, buy small quantities so that they will not sit on your shelf for a long time.

**Q:** What are the fruit acids commonly used and where are they derived from?

**A:** Common fruit acids used in cosmetic formulations and their common sources are the following: (1) Glycolic acid — sugar

cane, (2) Lactic acid — sour milk, beer, sauerkraut, pickles, (3)
Citric acid — citrus fruits, (4) Malic acid — unripened apples,
(5) Mandelic acid — extract of bitter almonds, (6) Tartaric acid
— fermented grapes.[9]

**Q:** What are the common acids incorporated in skin care products?
**A:** The common acids incorporated in skin care products found
over-the-counter are: AHAs (glycolic acid, lactic acid, mandelic
acid, benzilic acid), salicylic acid, citric acid, and ascorbic acid.
Common acids used in the doctor's office or incorporated in
prescription skin care products are: higher concentrations of
AHA's, trichloroacetic acid, tretinoin, and azelaic acid.

**Q:** What do you think of tretinoin (vitamin A derivative)?
**A:** Tretinoin is one of my first-line treatments for moderate to
severe acne. Tretinoin has also been shown to produce significant improvement in fine and coarse wrinkling, sallowness,
roughness of sun-damaged facial and arm skin. It has also been
shown to repair some changes from sun damage in the dermis,
increase the thickness of the epidermis (upper skin layer), enhance the skin blood supply, and bring about new collagen
deposition. Tretinoin has been demonstrated to reverse (or
maybe produce new changes that mimic a reversal) age-associ-
ated changes in tissue.[8]

The drug works but it is quite difficult to use because it may
cause peeling, dryness, and skin irritation. One needs to use
tretinoin sparingly and with caution not to use it too often if one
experiences some or all of the side effects that I have mentioned.
Tretinoin is now formulated in a less irritating and moisturizing
base. This formulation is indicated for the aging and sun-
damaged skin and not specifically for acne Each individual
responds quite differently from another, therefore, I tailor my
recommended regimen to the needs of each individual patient.
I follow every patient very closely in the beginning of his or her
treatment regimen and I modify the routine as we go along until
we reach a comfortable level of success. Remember: There is

not one recipe for good skin. What is good for your friend may not be exactly what is best for you.

**Q:** What do you think of formulations containing vitamin C?

**A:** I myself am using a facial cream containing vitamin C and I am using it twice a day. Once in the morning after washing my face with a 2% salicylic acid soap bar and another time is at night after washing my face with the 2% salicylic acid soap bar. In the short time that I had been using this new product, I am quite pleased with the results that I have obtained. First of all, I noticed my skin feels smoother and "shinier" (there is a nice glow on the surface) compared to the normal state of my skin prior to using this product. I also noticed some lightening of the patchy superficial dark discoloration on my face which is due to melasma (refer to chapters on The Aging Skin and Skin Discoloration). Third, I noticed my acne breakouts lessened.

Vitamin C, an acid commonly derived from fruits, is a natural acid. Changes in pH on the skin surface may alter the permeability of the skin to various substances. Acids in general, as we know, may cause irritancy of the skin surface, thus, a resultant exfoliation may occur. Vitamin C (L-ascorbic acid) in higher concentrations may cause varying degrees of skin irritancy. Ascorbic acid (vitamin C) stimulates collagen synthesis.[11,15] Ascorbic acid has been shown to have some protective effects from the sun.[12,19] Remember: It is not a sunscreen. Ascorbic acid also has been shown to improve some superficial sun damage and possibly prevent tumor formation.

I am quite impressed with the results that I have observed with the use of a cream containing Vitamin C and I am looking forward to learning more about the beneficial effects of this natural acid on our skin.

**Q:** What do you think of formulations containing Vitamin E (alpha tocopherol)?

**A:** The biological functions of vitamin E (alpha tocopherol) are not fully established. Some of its benefits were shown in animal studies. These benefits may include the prevention of skin cancer formation. However, these results are not definitely established in humans.

**Q:** What do you think of EGF (Epidermal Growth Factor)?

**A:** I have used a new skin cream containing EGF over a limited period. EGF in this particular skin cream is combined with ingredients that are known to have an emollient or moisturizing effect on the skin. I have observed over this limited period that it did moisturize my skin but I noticed further enlargement of several already prominent sebaceous or oil glands as well as enlargement of small existing milial cysts on my face. Cosmetically, I am concerned with these results over a short period of application so I immediately stopped its use. I would like to see a positive use of EGF and other growth factors in wound healing and skin injuries after thorough confirmation with clinical trials.

**Q:** What are the common nutritional deficiencies and their skin manifestations?

**A:** The following is a summary of common nutritional deficiencies and their skin manifestations (I included experimental findings in animals because it is extremely difficult for certain experiments to be conducted in human subjects. The animal findings may be relevant to the human species. If not, you may take it as an interesting thought to ponder upon.):

| Nutritional Deficiency | Skin Manifestation |
| --- | --- |
| Riboflavin (vitamin B$_2$) | Inflammation at the corners of the mouth, seborrheic dermatitis around the nose and scrotum, inflammation of the tongue, changes in the cornea of the eye. |
| Niacin (nicotinic acid) | Pellagra or darkened, thickened scaly eruption in light exposed areas, inflammation of the tongue, diarrhea, mental disturbances. |
| Folic acid | Inflammation of the lips, inflammation of the tongue, sores in the mouth, discoloration and seborrheic dermatitis on the genital area. |

| Nutritional Deficiency | Skin Manifestation |
|---|---|
| Panthotenic acid | No spontaneous deficiencies occur in humans. Loss of hair color is produced in mice, hair loss is produced in dogs, dermatitis in swine, and dermatitis with poor feathering in chicks.[21] A healthy anecdote: Marvin, a patient of mine who comes in regularly every year for his complete skin examination brought me a bottle of vitamins (Sundown®) that he has been taking in the past six months. These vitamins contain 500 mg panthotenic acid. After my complete examination, I noted that hairs are growing in Marvin's bald spot on the crown of his head! (This is one reason why I included the animal studies that may or may not be relevant to humans.) |
| Biotin | Acquired biotin deficiency is rare in humans because it is synthesized in the intestines by bacteria, but may occur from excess intake of raw egg or when intestinal bacteria is altered. Experimental deficiencies in humans led to thinning of the surface of the tongue, dermatitis, dry skin, grayness of the lining of the mouth. |
| Vitamin $B_{12}$ (cyanocobalamine) | Dark discoloration of the arms, hands and legs. |
| Vitamin E | No specific effects have been shown in humans. Hemorrhage and swelling under the skin has been shown in chicks. In premature infants, redness, seborrheic changes, dryness, and loss of skin color have been ascribed to vitamin E deficiency. |
| Vitamin K | Impaired blood clotting and skin hemorrhage. |
| Magnesium | There are no dermatologic manifestations in clinical human magnesium deficiency. In rats, skin changes include redness, swelling, hair loss and thickened growths on the skin. In gerbils, hair loss was noted.[17] |
| Iron | Nail abnormalities, inflammation of the corners of the mouth, inflammation of the tongue, ulcers in the mouth, susceptibility to yeast infections on the skin and mucous membranes. Word of caution: Iron overload causes darkening and extreme dryness with scaling of the skin. |
| Potassium | No definite skin changes in humans. In rats, deficiency causes hair loss. In mice, it causes a lusterless coat and a dry scaly tail. |

| Nutritional Deficiency | Skin Manifestation |
|---|---|
| Selenium | Selenium, like vitamin E has been shown to inhibit initiation of skin cancer by acting as an antioxidant scavenger. In one human family, selenium deficiency was associated with hair loss, and thin and abnormal nails. |
| Protein–Energy Malnutrition (PEM) | Dryness, thinning of the skin, large areas of skin darkening, thickening of the surface of the skin, peeling, brittle nails, fragile hair, loss of hair color. Note: Hair can be utilized to determine the onset of PEM by measuring the distance of the abnormality from the hair root and considering the rate of hair growth (refer to chapter on The Hair). |
| Amino acid deficiency | Generalized amino acid deficiency in humans is associated with necrosis of the upper skin layer, blistering, and loss of hair. Tryptophan (one form of amino acid) deficiency in rat or guinea pig is associated with hair loss.[17] |
| Zinc | Patients with zinc deficiency have been shown to be prone to bacterial and yeast infections. In rats, significant depression of cellular immunity had been demonstrated. In humans, zinc had been demonstrated to play a major role in the proliferation of lymphocytes (lymphocytes are regulators of immunity). Skin manifestations in cattle include hair loss, skin infections, and thickened skin growths.[13] |
| Copper | Copper is an essential micronutrient required in the formation of important enzymes. Skin-related consequences of copper deficiency in certain enzymes include failure of pigmentation and hair abnormality. Note: The copper content of sweat is quite high and excessive sweating may lead to a significant loss of copper. Some workers have postulated that the amount of copper absorbed into the skin from copper bracelets can be sufficient to have some effect on the arthritic process.[6] |

Word of caution: Some vitamin preparations may be more effective than others. Allergic skin reaction may result with certain vitamins, minerals, or additives.

**Q:** I turn red easily when I am in the sun. How do I protect my face?

**A:** You probably have rosacea (refer to Rosacea chapter) or you have Type I or Type II skin (refer to Skin Cancer chapter). Before going into the sun, wash your face with a gentle soap-free cleanser or a mild soap that is not too drying to the skin. Rinse with cool to tepid water. Then apply a sunscreen with a moisturizing base. The choice of sunscreen base preparation is very important because certain sunscreens can cause a burning sensation or irritation on your skin, usually caused by an alcohol base in the sunscreen. You may apply your make-up after you apply your sunscreen. Certain make-up and moisturizer preparations are combined with a sunscreen. Make sure that you pick a combined preparation with an SPF 15.

**Q:** I have acne that I want to cover up. What do I do?

**A:** First, wash your face with a mild soap or a medicated face wash prescribed for you. If you have skin dryness, apply a non-comedogenic moisturizer. If there is no remarkable dryness, apply any topical medication prescribed for you. If you are going out in the sun, apply an oil-free sunscreen after washing your face.

After doing any of the above, you may apply an oil-free or water-based make-up. Then apply your eye make-up and lipstick.

Wash your face again at night with a mild soap or medicated face wash. Then apply the acne medication prescribed for you.

Discolorations due to acne may be camouflaged with make-up. Consult a make-up artist regarding proper camouflage if you are unable to accomplish it on your own by using a concealer or a good make-up base. Word of caution: The concealer or make-up base you are using should be non-comedogenic in order to prevent further breakouts.

**Q:** How do I find the right make-up base that will not make me break out?

**A:** This may be a tough job and may require some trial and error until you find the right one. There is a sulfur-based medication that is tinted which can serve as a base for you. Ask your dermatologist about this. As far as regular make-up is concerned, a good way to start is to scout the make-up counters in the stores. Find a product that is non-comedogenic and allergy tested, preferably on human beings. If you can get a tester that will last for at least a couple of weeks with everyday use, great! It may take at least two weeks for a delayed reaction to occur on your skin. You will also find out if this product is the right color or is cosmetically acceptable to you. If there are no testers available, then you must invest money to try out this new product. A good rule is to try out new cosmetics, one product at a time, for at least two weeks apart or longer because it takes time to develop a delayed reaction to a product. This will help you determine whether the product is suitable for you and it will be easier to pinpoint or eliminate any problems.

Due to the above reasons, I, myself, had spent much money and thrown out many cosmetics that I had purchased. I finally came to the conclusion that there is nothing better than clear skin and looking natural. I use cosmetics to enhance or to add some color to my appearance. I would rather have clear skin without much make-up than suffer breakouts caused by make-up use.

Sometimes we get in a situation where a person uses a lot of make-up to conceal broken-out skin and claims that her breakout does not seem to get better no matter what she does to take care or treat her skin. This is quite a disarming situation. This person needs guidance from an expert who has compassion and understanding. Dermatologic guidance and treatment and thorough step-by-step coaching is necessary to get out of this cosmetic and psychological dilemma.

ta.

### Ligaya On . . . Life

*There is a very important lesson that I learned when my father passed away. I worked so hard to become what I am and he did not even see me in my doctor's coat because he passed on before his visitor's visa was approved. I learned to live life to the fullest and be grateful for its graces.*

**Q:** Is one make-up brand better than another?

**A:** An individual with trouble-free skin can usually use many of the over-the-counter make-up brands. However, make-up manufacturers may produce different quality make-up. I have thrown out several lip liners and eyeliners that have dried out and do not line properly.

The choice of the right color is another important factor in make-up. You must realize that the color you see on the counter may not reproduce the way it appears when applied to your skin. This is particularly true with lipstick and blush.

The consistency of make-up is also very important. Some may feel greasy, may not absorb well, or may just not feel good or stay right on the skin.

**Q:** Is scrubbing good for the skin?

**A:** The answer is no. Scrubbing is a form of trauma to the skin. Whenever you traumatize the skin, an inflammatory reaction follows and this may leave skin discoloration or cause roughness. You may wash your face with a soft washcloth or soft sponge but I highly recommend using your bare hands. Be sure to wash the washcloth and sponge with soap after each use and replace them regularly in order to avoid bacterial or fungal build-up.

I also do not recommend the use of harsh brushes for the rest of the body for the same reason stated above. The use of mild exfoliants in the form of a soap, lotion, or cream (for example, 2% salicyclic acid soap, AHA, or vitamin C formulation) is preferable over the use of "loofah" scrubs. Your skin will naturally shed and the subsequent application of a moisturizer will smooth out the surface. Most of the mild exfoliant creams or lotions are already combined with a moisturizing base, and you may not need to use an added moisturizer in this particular situation.

**Q:** Is there such a thing as a pore minimizer?

**A:** Not exactly. Some individuals have naturally more prominent pores compared to others. However, in the case of clogged pores, when you use Retin A®, Differin,® or Azelex® for example, some of those plugs may loosen up and exfoliate. Other acid exfoliants like AHAs and salicyclic acid are similarly aimed to loosen up and remove those follicular plugs. Therefore, emptying the clogged pores has a beneficial effect. Pores that are not clogged will not get smaller. Applying a moisturizer on the general skin surface will enhance the smooth appearance of the skin.

**Q:** Do I need a skin astringent and toner?

**A:** What you basically need is to clean the skin surface of the dead cell build-up, surface dirt, and skin oil or sebum build-up. This can be accomplished by a mild soap and water, a soap-free cleanser, a mild exfoliant like AHA wash, cream, lotion, or gel or salicylic acid soap. You need to seal in some moisture on the skin surface to prevent dryness, itching, and flaking after any of these treatments. I recommend you select a non-comedogenic and hypoallergenic moisturizer for this purpose (refer to questions on: What are the common active ingredients in moisturizers? and How do I keep my skin nice and smooth?).

Astringents do not reduce the rate of oil production by our oil glands under the surface of the skin. Why spend more money with expensive astringents if you can achieve the same results with soap and water or soap-free cleansers? Alcohol has a drying effect on the skin surface and causes skin surface moisture loss. It does not stop oil production by the oil glands.

**Q:** I developed a terrible itch all of a sudden. What can I do?

**A:** First, examine your body in front of the mirror and see if there is any redness, discoloration, roughness, or blotchiness anywhere. If you see any of the above and the symptoms persist over 24 hours despite your regular moisturizing daily routine, I recommend that you see a dermatologist or physician as soon as possible because you will save a lot of anguish, time, and money in the long run the sooner this problem is controlled or cured.

If you do not see any rash, try to moisturize your skin on a regular daily or twice a day basis. You may purchase a moisturizer over the counter containing camphor and/or phenol like

Sarna® lotion if your regular moisturizer does not work. Try taking an antihistamine such as diphenhydramine (available over the counter) at bedtime. Be careful with the use of some antihistamines because one of their most common side effects is drowsiness. Avoid these when driving or using all machinery.

Avoid using over-the-counter salves containing lanocaine or any of the other "-caine" preparations. These are known to have a great potential to sensitize your skin. In other words, they may cause an allergic reaction, adding a rash and more itching to your problem.

**Q:** I plan to go to the beach, what is the best way for me to use a sunscreen?

**A:** Apply a water-resistant SPF 15 sunscreen or higher an hour prior to arriving at the beach. Make sure that you apply this to the entire skin surface that will be exposed to the sun. Do not forget areas like your ears, behind your ears, underneath your eyes, nose, lips, and even your bald spots. Certain sunscreen preparations applied on the forehead and above the eyes may cause a burning sensation in your eyes when you start to sweat. You can remedy this by skipping the sunscreen on these areas and by wearing a visor or hat. You may apply the sunscreen on this area and wear a headband to stop the sweat from dripping down into your eyes. This is the reason professional tennis players wear headbands.

**Q:** What does SPF in a sunscreen mean?

**A:** SPF or sun protection factor is a quantitative measure of the effectiveness of a sunscreen. It is based on the ultraviolet light-absorbing properties of the active ingredient or ingredients of the sunscreen formulation:

$$SPF = \frac{MED \text{ (minimum erythema dose) of the sunscreen-protected skin}}{MED \text{ (minimum erythema dose) of the non-protected skin}}$$

SPF is the ratio of the least amount of ultraviolet energy (MED) required to produce a minimal redness reaction through a sunscreen product film to the amount of energy required to produce the same amount of redness without the sunscreen.[14] In other words, a sunscreen with an SPF 8 will theoretically protect you 8 times longer prior to developing minimal skin redness from the sun versus not using a sunscreen at all. These tests are done with an indoor solar stimulator and the SPF value when measured under direct sunlight may not be the same value with the SPF measured with an indoor solar stimulator. For example, an SPF 15 measured with an indoor solar stimulator for a product may measure SPF 12 when measured outdoors under direct sunlight.

**Q:** What commercial sunscreen protects me the most from ultraviolet light?

**A:** The following sunscreen components protect you from UVA:
   parsol
   benzophenones

The following sunscreen components protect you from UVB:
   PABA
   PABA esters
   benzophenones
   cinnamates
   salicylates
   anthralinates

The following sunscreen components protect you from both UVA and UVB:
   titanium dioxide — 5% to 20%
   talc or magnesium silicate
   magnesium oxide
   zinc oxide
   kaolin
   ferric chloride
   ichthyol or ichthammol[14]

The sunscreen base is also very important. Water-based sunscreens generally need to be reapplied more frequently as compared to oil-based sunscreens because water-based products tend to wash off more easily. However, I recommend the use of water-based products for certain skin conditions like acne.

Some individuals may be allergic to certain ingredients like PABA. In this case, this particular ingredient must be avoided.

As you can see, an educated consumer really needs to read the labels of sunscreens on the market. A combination sunscreen (offers UVA and UVB protection) with the right concentration of components is better than one with a single agent.

Realistically, there is no total sunblock unless you use physical sun protection like the use of a wide brim hat or umbrella and protective clothing in addition to sunscreen with an SPF 15 or higher. Some protection is better than no protection. Pick your sunscreen based on the above ingredients if you can, otherwise, at least pick a number 15 or higher sunscreen. Reapply your sunscreen every couple of hours. Use other protective covering like clothing or hat to provide additional protection.

You can enjoy the outdoors. Now, you have the medication and the knowledge to protect yourself. Hopefully, in the next century, due to the current knowledge and medications available to us, we will see less premature wrinkling and sun-related skin diseases.

**Q:**   What is the difference between UVB (ultra violet B) and UVA (ultra violet A) effects on the skin?

**A:**   UVB and UVA represent two spectra of light wavelengths that have been shown to have the most harmful effects on the skin and cause skin diseases.

UVA causes the tanning reaction and the sunburn or redness reaction (sunburn producing capacity is weaker than UVB). UVA-induced redness is seen soon after exposure to sun which is within the first 12 hours. UVA is usually involved in sun-related allergic or toxic reactions.

UVB is the principal cause of the sunburn reaction which may lead to swelling and blistering. The redness is most prominent between 15 to 24 hours after exposure. UVB is more effective compared to UVA in causing the tanning reaction.

Both UVA and UVB can cause redness or sunburn and tanning but the amount of UVA energy required to produce these effects is much higher than the amount of UVB energy. The amount of solar UVA reaching the earth's surface is about 10 times greater than that of UVB.

The effects of UVA and UVB add up together.

Repeated UVA and UVB exposure can bring about permanent changes and damage to the skin. These effects occur following the first exposures in early life and are cumulative. The magnitude and variety of the effects depend on whether or not susceptible individuals have used sun protection throughout life and their natural defense mechanisms (refer to skin types in chapter on Skin Cancer).

Various UVA and UVB effects on the skin include the following:

1. Blood vessel effects — persistent redness, prominence of small blood vessels referred to as telangiectasia, or "weather beaten" face.
2. Skin cell effects — precancerous changes, skin cancer.
3. Skin pigment cell effects — freckles, solar lentigines, melanoma skin cancer.
4. Changes in the dermis which is right below the upper skin layer — wrinkling, roughening, yellowing, and thinning of the skin (leads to easy bruising).[14]

**Q:** What is a laser?

**A:** The word laser means Light Amplification by the Stimulated Emission of Radiation. Laser is a form of light but it differs from sunlight because it is of a single wavelength. This means that you can not form a rainbow out of a laser (if you recall your science experiment on how a rainbow is formed). Laser light is coherent, meaning the waves of energy are in phase with each other. Laser light is also collimated, meaning that the laser beam waves are parallel, producing a narrow and very straight beam that can be propagated for long distances.

**Q:**  What are the common types of LASERs that are being used?

**A:**  Common types of lasers are the following: (1) Carbon dioxide laser, (2) Argon laser, (3) Neodynium: Yag, (4) Excimer, (5) Metal vapor, (6) Tunable dye lasers or pulsed dye lasers, (7) Photodynamic therapy, (8) Ruby, (9) Helium-Neon. Your physician will determine which laser is appropriate to use for your particular condition.

**Q:**  What are collagen injections?

**A:**  There are three available forms of injectable collagen approved by the FDA at present. These include Zyderm I, Zyderm II and Zyplast. Zyderm collagen is derived from cowhide which undergoes a method of purification and sterilization. Zyplast collagen is bovine dermal collagen cross-linked by glutaraldehyde. A skin testing is necessary prior to collagen injection. Side effects of collagen injections include: bruising, bacterial infections, activation of herpes simplex within areas injected, local necrosis of skin, partial vision loss (very rare occurrence), swelling, itching, redness, hypersensitivity reaction (most of these reactions subside within a year but some may persist longer than two years). Some physicians have speculated that exposure to injectable collagen puts patients at risk of developing autoimmune disease. A panel of rheumatologist and immunologists reexamined the knowledge on autoimmune disease and the immune response to bovine dermal collagen. They concluded that current data did not support the suggestion that xenogenic dermal collagen exposure could precipitate autoimmune disease in humans or other species.[10] Personally, I decided to stop giving injectable collagen for deep lines to my patients because of the high cost of collagen and the relatively short lifespan of the desired cosmetic results.

**Q:**  What is liposuction?

**A:**  Liposuction is a surgical procedure that removes localized areas of fat accumulation that are resistant to exercise and diet. It is not a treatment for surface skin irregularities like cellulite. It is

ᘒᘒ

## Ligaya On . . . Synchronicity

*Synchronicity is the way Nature hands a presnt. To recognize it is to commune with Nature. An example of synchronicity: I needed a publisher and I met a friend who put me in touch with her client who is a publisher. I called this publisher and she turned out to be an old friend of mine who I had lost touch with. I did not realize that she was in the publishing business and she did not know that I write. She read my manuscript and fell in love with it!*

not a treatment for obesity. The response of fat cells to diet and exercise varies in different anatomic regions of the body.[1] Those fat cells that require near starvation before reducing their volume are found in the abdomen and flanks of men and in the thighs and hips of women. It has been theorized that the number of fat cells is fixed at puberty. Unless the individual becomes extremely obese, the number of fat cells remain the same. Weight gain or loss after puberty depends on the increase in volume and size of the fat cells. These concepts are the basis of the theory of liposuction that the removal of resistant cells produces a permanent decrease in the size and number of localized areas of fatty tissue.[7]

**Q:**  What is hair transplant surgery?

**A:**  Hair transplant surgery is the removal of hair plugs from one area of the scalp and "planting" these hair plugs to the bald area of the scalp. This procedure is based on the principle that the hair follicle retains its own characteristics. Therefore, since the hair follicles at the occipital region (back of the scalp) are less likely to be affected by the balding tendency in male-pattern baldness, one can transplant these hair follicles to the frontal scalp (the front area of the scalp where you usually notice male-pattern baldness). They will not be affected by the balding tendency on the frontal part of the scalp.

# Part V

# Dr. Buchbinder's Personal Keys to Beauty

My Personal Beauty Routines

Postscript

.

# Chapter 28

# My Personal Beauty Routines

**Dr. Buchbinder's Skin Care Routine and Experiences in Skin Care Before She Was 20: Traditions and Old Routines May Still Be Reliable**

I am one of those teenagers who was blessed with beautiful Oriental skin and thick long, straight black hair. Not only that, I was also one of those kids who devoured a chocolate bar and ate a pint of ice cream for snacks and always stayed below 100 pounds. For me skin care was real simple then. I used whatever shampoo was sitting on the shower counter and whatever soap my mother brought home from the supermarket. I preferred then a conditioning shampoo because it was too much trouble for me to shampoo my hair, rinse, apply a hair conditioner, and rinse again. I got out of the shower, combed my hair, put on my clothes and off I went! No make-up, no powder, and no other salves on my skin.

I stayed in a girl's dormitory from age 12 because I studied in the nation's capital. This was a great opportunity for me. I was away on a scholarship wherein everything was paid for by the Philippine government. We were even provided some pocket money. I lived and socialized practically with the same group of girls and boys for 5

&

## Ligaya On . . . Power

*Many times we feel overwhelmed of work. Yes! There is a lot of work to be done. Helpful hint: Make a DECISION. Set your priorities. Take a bite of the deli platter systematically. If you hate one item, toss it out! If you hate two items, toss them out. If you hate the whole platter, throw the whole thing out. Do not get sick by forcing yourself to eat a bad platter. You can create your own platter. Once the DECISION is clear, the right action will follow. There is no such thing as a wrong decision. What matters is you made one and followed it through with what you think is appropriate action. You may or may not like the results. If not, make another decision and aim for a different result. This is what life is all about. Making small and big decisions and learning from their outcomes. This is one secret to gain personal power.*

years. Of course we girls ventured to meet other boys from other schools whenever we could.

The dormitory was the place where we learned skin care. The only doctor we saw was the one at the school clinic who had a fixed recipe for fever of any kind. We all had a baggage of superstitions, myths, and empirical facts handed down to us from our ancestors to our parents. We were all scholars, so we "knew" what was right for us. Emilia had a ritual of painstakingly rubbing Jergen's lotion all over her body when she got out of the shower every single day. Her skin did look smooth and shiny. Lillian used to go through jars of Esoterica applied over her entire face in the morning and at bedtime. I never really noticed a difference on her skin but she swore by it. Gloria used to go for a hot oil treatment on her scalp once a month. None of us really noticed a difference but if it made her feel good, it was cool. Ellen used to go to bed with a white face every single night. She applied Clearasil regularly to treat her acne. She had a lot of pimples. (I saw Ellen as an adult lately and I did not notice any remarkable acne scars on her face). Several girls with dandruff were using Head and Shoulders shampoo. I used it once in a while. Some girls used a solid rock of alum (wetting it prior to rubbing the underarms) for their deodorant. Jean applied a hydrocortisone cream for a few days whenever she got an insect bite. We shared her emergency cream whenever we got bit. We helped each other whenever one got the head lice. We would take turns to sit and pick out the nits and used a fine comb to get rid of the crawling adult lice. Gross? This is a common practice in the Orient amongst friends and family. We had an isolation room for the measles, chickenpox, or any other contagious illness, otherwise we got confined in the infirmary. (I recently picked up a bar of alum from a spa in Bangkok and I am using it now for my deodorant. It solved my problem of clothes staining from antiperspirants. A bar will last me at least for six months).

## Dr. Buchbinder' Skin Care Routine Before 40: I Needed a Little Extra and I Knew More About Skin Care

I started breaking out with mild adult acne after I was 20. Early on, I never really bothered with skin care. I still followed my simple teenage routine. In fact, my husband still dreams of me in medical school at 25 without make-up and with long, straight hair. Then I moved to New York City at 27. Lots of adjustments to be made, completely different environment, new responsibilities, and merging into a whole new culture. What does a 27 year-old girl without any make-up do as she passes the make-up department of Bloomingdale's? I really did not intend to do anything, but the make-up artist just happened to give a free make-over that afternoon and she graciously offered to do this on me! Well, all this for free — why not? I came home that day so delighted to show my "improved" appearance to my husband and his face just about dropped! This expression reminded me of his reaction when I showed up on the day of our wedding with my face made up and my long hair combed up in a double French braid. He had specifically asked me to promise him that I would not wear any make-up and would wear my hair down for our wedding.

Do I really listen to my husband, despite the fact that he is also a dermatologist, as far as skin care is concerned? I do like to hear his reassurance and his suggestions, but to me skin care is as personal as brushing my teeth. I do what I feel and what I think is right for me, after hearing his excellent suggestions.

After I gave birth to my first child at the age of 32, my skin and body underwent tremendous changes. During the last trimester of pregnancy, I developed those unsightly bluish-purple bags underneath my eyes. I discussed this with my plastic surgeon Danny (I call him by his first name because he happens to be one of our dear friends) and he told me that there is now a trans-conjunctival procedure wherein he can remove the enlarged fat tissue causing the bags by cutting in the conjunctiva. There is no cutting on the exposed skin surface therefore there are no scars. I was very nervous because this was my first plastic surgical procedure. I have to admit that without my husband's under-standing, it would have been more difficult. He gave me his support despite not understanding his "perfect" wife's need for plastic surgery. I went into surgery two weeks after I delivered my baby boy, stayed overnight in his recovery room, and the next morning went home to have breakfast with my family. What a cinch!

Despite all these changes, I pretty much stayed with a very simple skin care routine. My skin type remained normal to slightly oily on the T-zone. I washed my face two times a day with 2% salicylic acid soap bar and rinsed with tepid water, I applied a moisturizer with an SPF 15 on my face and a regular moisturizer on my body (contains dimethicone, petrolatum and glycerine as active ingredients) in the morning, and applied 0.05% tretinoin cream on my face every other night for my mild adult acne. I tried AHAs in multiple different formulations and a multitude of other moisturizers from the sample closet in my office but I found that the things I used were sufficient for my skin. I applied the blush directly on my cheeks, outlined my lips with a lip liner, applied my lipstick, once in a while applied an eye liner and that was it!

## Dr. Buchbinder's Skin Care Routine After 40: I Need to Do Something Different to Turn the Aging Clock Backwards!

We went on a holiday trip to the Orient with our good friends Dena and Danny. As we were sitting lazily under an umbrella on the beach, I mentioned how I was really bothered by my abdominal bulge. My husband started reassuring me in the background how I do not need any procedure for this area. I told Danny that we will seriously talk about it when we get back to Boca Raton. In the meantime, down the white sand beach of Phuket, Thailand is an oriental woman of about 30 in her bikini, doing some body contortions. She seemed to be saluting the sun at the same time. This woman was fascinating because she had the flattest abdomen and tiptop body shape from the distance. Dena and I walked towards her to take a closer look and I saw stretch marks all over her upper thighs and abdomen despite her taut skin (as a dermatologist, this suggested to me that she must have been heavier in these areas at some point). Dena told me that she must be doing some kind of yoga postures. Dena told me that she knew where yoga classes are held at home. I told Danny that I will look into this yoga as soon as we get home and that I will hold off on the liposuction and abdominoplasty.

As soon as we got back, I found out that I can go for Hatha yoga classes three times a week in the evenings and on Saturday morning. This changed Ligaya at 41! Every month after I started, I saw incredible changes on my body and along with it are changes to my total persona. Patients who have not seen me for a year almost do not recognize their doctor. I changed my hair style. I added translucent powder, bronzing powder, brushed my eyebrows with a dark brown color, and regularly used an eyeliner. I even tease my hair at the root and gently comb it over and fix it with a light hairspray to keep it up the whole day (I lost about half the thickness of my hair because I follow the hair thinning tendency that runs in my family). I also apply a dark brown color rinse once every five weeks to cover some gray hair. This year, I got hold of an ascorbic acid cream that does a phenomenal job of giving me smoother, shinier, and less acne-prone skin! There are several of these products in the market but one particular formulation better suited my sensitive, acne-prone skin. At least I have postponed my tummy tuck for now and everything that I am doing seems to be working well at this time. Never say never — but maybe puts one in a flexible position!

A regular work day for me now starts around 5 o'clock in the morning with 1-1/2 hours of Hatha yoga, a cup of Longjing tea (got these tea bags from Hong Kong) with a piece of toast with jelly. I get my two children ready for school, go to work, eat my bagged lunch, back to work, take care of the kids after school, cook dinner, put the kids to bed and start working on my projects until close to midnight. Five hours of sleep is all I need and I am truly energized, ready for a full day of work after my Hatha yoga routine.

I honestly believe that turning back or slowing down the aging clock is possible to a certain point. Always keep an open mind. It entails a tremendous commitment and total discipline which transcends the physical. One needs to integrate the body, mind, and spirit. Once it is integrated, one radiates that light that shines around and affects everything in sight, consciously or subliminally. It is very difficult to intentionally change what and who is around you, but once you have changed, everything molds right into your being.

# Chapter 29

# Postscript

As I look across the calm water I see a moving bright light coming towards me. I search for the source. I see a hanging piece of tin across the bay, moving with the wind. I look up and see the bright morning sun. I realize that the moving light was a reflection of the sun as it shines on the piece of tin hanging out there. The calm water's surface is in turn reflecting the bright light onto me.

Think of the tin as the mirror that we look at everyday. Imagine you as the sun reflecting your own light. YOU are the first person to perceive your own light. Imagine your mind as the water on the bay.

Your perception will be influenced by the state of your mind as the reflection of the sun will be affected by the calmness or the roughness of the water on the bay. Other people's perception of you will be influenced by the state of their mind.

As we say — beauty is relative. There is a mate for every soul.

There are billions of mirrors that reflect your persona and their perception of you will be influenced by the state of each individual's mind. Each time you change your persona, your reflection will be changed on these billions of mirrors.

Do you really know how the mirror of your soulmate should reflect you? We can only speculate. Speculations are not exact.

On my part, I choose to trust my basic guts or instinct. By doing this, I go down to my very core. There are no mirrors when I go by my guts because I bypass the mirror of my mind. I trust that my soulmate will also go by his basic guts thereby bypassing his mirror in his mind. This way, we judge our essence.

*"Mirror, mirror on the wall, who is the fairest of us all?*
*. . . Thou art the fairest since thou beholdest."*

# Part VI _____

# Glossary

*  **Acne.**  An inflammatory disorder of the oil glands that causes pimples.
*  **Acid.**  pH ("pouvoire Hydrogene") below 7. Turns blue litmus paper pink. May cause skin irritation, peeling, or burning.
*  **Adapalene.**  New generation of topical retinoid.
*  **AHA.**  Alpha hydroxy acid which commonly includes glycolic acid, lactic acid, mandelic acid and benzilic acid.
*  **Alkali.**  Of pH ("pouvoire Hydrogene") above 7. Turns pink litmus paper blue. May cause skin irritation.
*  **Allergen.**  Incitant of altered reactivity (allergy).
*  **Alopecia.**  Loss of hair.
*  **Alopecia areata.**  Patchy hair loss not due to an infectious process.
*  **Anagen.**  Growing stage in the hair growth cycle.
*  **Androgen.**  Hormone that stimulates the activity of the accessory sex organs of the male.
*  **Androgenic alopecia.**  Male or female pattern baldness.
*  **Antihistamine.**  Antagonize or neutralize the action of histamine or inhibit its production in the body.
*  **Ascorbic acid.**  Vitamin C.
*  **Catagen.**  Transitional stage between growing and resting in the hair growth cycle.
*  **Carcinogenic.**  Cancer promoting.

- **Comedogenic.** The tendency to cause blackheads upon application on the skin surface.
- **Cryosurgery.** Surgery with use of decreased temperature.
- **Cystic acne.** Scarring form of acne.
- **Dermis.** The middle layer of the skin.
- **Eczema.** Derived from the Greek word "ekzein" meaning "to boil out" or "to effervesce."
- **EGF.** Epidermal growth factor. It is a factor contained in tissue or fluid that stimulates an increase in the number or proliferation of skin cells.
- **Electrosurgery.** The use of electricity in surgery.
- **Epidermis.** The outermost layer of the skin.
- **Exclamatory pointed hair.** The shape of hair like an exclamation mark (!) typically found in alopecia areata.
- **Exfoliate.** Shed the uppermost skin layer.
- **Goeckerman regimen.** Treatment for psoriasis consiting of tar and ultraviolet light.
- **Group A beta-hemolytic Streptococcus.** Strain of Streptococcus bacteria that may cause an acute kidney infection.
- **HPV.** Human Papilloma Virus which cause warts.
- **Herpes zoster.** Shingles.
- **Impetigo.** Skin infection usually due to *Staphylococcus* or *Streptococcus* bacteria.
- **Keratinocytes.** Skin cells.
- **Laser.** Light amplification by stimulated emission of radiation.
- **Lentigo.** Freckle or "liver spot."
- **Melanocyte.** Pigment cell of the skin.
- **Melasma.** Mask of pregnancy.
- **Melanosomes.** Pigment granules produced by melanocytes.
- **Nevus flammeus.** Port-wine stain.
- **Oral Candidiasis.** "Thrush" or yeast infection of the mouth.
- **PABA.** Para-aminobenzoic acid. Found in sunscreen.
- **Paronychia.** Inflammation of the nail fold.
- **Pruritus.** Itching.
- **Pseudofolliculitis.** Ingrown hair.
- **Psoriasis.** Skin disease characterized by red, dry, scaly patches of various sizes.

🙰 **Retinoid.** Vitamin A derivative.

🙰 **Retinoid analog.** Not a true vitamin A derivative but has chemical properties similar to a vitamin A derivative.

🙰 **Rosacea.** Disorder of the face characterized by redness, telangiectasia, and acne-like breakouts.

🙰 **Sebaceous glands.** Oil-producing glands.

🙰 **Seborrheic dermatitis.** Dandruff. Characterized by build-up of oily scales over reddened or pink skin.

🙰 **Striae.** Stretch marks.

🙰 **Sulzberger's formula.** 2 tablespoons olive oil + large glass of milk + tepid bathwater.

🙰 **Telangiectasia.** Dilated blood vessel in the skin.

🙰 **Telogen.** Resting stage in the hair growth cycle.

🙰 **Telogen effluvium.** Early and excessive loss of normal hairs.

🙰 **Tinea versicolor.** Superficial fungus infection causing white, pink or brown spots.

🙰 **Tinea cruris.** Jock itch.

🙰 **Tocopherol.** Vitamin E.

🙰 **Tretinoin.** Vitamin A derivative. A retinoid.

🙰 **UVA.** Ultra violet A.

🙰 **UVB.** Ultra violet B.

🙰 **Vitiligo.** White patches due to loss of skin pigment.

# Bibliography

[1] Arner, P. (1984) Site differences in human subcutaneous tissue metabolism in obesity. *Aesthetic Plast. Surg.* 8:13–17.

[2] Arnold, H.L., Odom, R.B. and James, W.D. (1990) *Andrews' Diseases of the Skin*, 8th ed., Philadelphia, W. B. Saunders Company, 6:89–130; 33:879.

[3] Bergfeld, W.F. (1992) Hair Disorders. In *Dermatology*. Moschella, S.L. and Hurley, H.J. (eds.), 3rd ed., Philadelphia, W. B. Saunders Company, 61:1451–1560.

[4] Bickers, D.R. (1991) Photosensitization by Porphyrins. In *Physiology, Biochemistry, and Molecular Biology of the Skin*. Goldsmith, L.A. (ed.), 2nd ed., New York, Oxford University Press, 35:957–975.

[5] Brody, H.J. (1989) The art of chemical peeling. *J Dermatol. Surg. Oncol.* 15:918–921.

[6] Danks, D.M. (1991) Copper deficiency and the skin. In *Physiology, Biochemistry, and Molecular Biology of the Skin*. Goldsmith. L.A. (ed.), 2nd ed., New York, Oxford University Press, 51:1351–1361.

[7] Dolsky, R.L. (1992) Current concepts and techniques in liposuction surgery. In *Dermatology*. Moschella, S.L. and Hurley, H.J. (eds.), 3rd ed., Philadelphia, W. B. Saunders Company, 97:2462–2470.

[8] Gilchrist, B.A. (1991) Physiology and pathophysiology of aging skin. In *Physiology, Biochemistry, and Molecular Biology of the Skin*. Goldsmith, L.A. (ed.), 2nd ed., New York, Oxford University Press, 54:1425–1444.

[9] Jackson, E.M. (Sept 1996) Using an acid on your face: What deos it really mean? *Cosmetic Dermatol.*, 9:47–48.

[10] Klein, A.W. (1992) Injectable collagen. In *Dermatology*. Moschella, S.L. and Hurley, H.J. (eds.), 3rd ed., Philadelphia, W. B. Saunders Company, 96:2455–2461.

[11] Murad, S., Grove, D., Lindberg, K.A., Reynolds, G., Sivarajah, A. and Pinnell, S.R. (1981) Regulation of collagen synthesis by ascorbic acid. *Proc. Natl. Acad. Sci. U.S.A.* 78:2879–2882.

[12] Nakamura, T., Pinnell, S.R. and Streilein, J.W. (April 1995) Antioxidants can reverse the deleterious effects of ultraviolet UVB radiation on cutaneous immunity. *J. of Invest. Dermatol.*, 104:600.

[13] Neldner, K.H. (1991) The biochemistry and physiology of zinc metabolism. In *Physiology, Biochemistry, and Molecular Biology of the Skin*. Goldsmith, L.A. (ed.), 2nd ed., New York, Oxford University Press, 50:1329–1349.

[14] Pathak, M.A. and Fitzpatrick, T.B. (1993). Preventive treatment of sunburn, dermatoheliosis, and skin cancer with sun-protective agents. In *Dermatology in General Medicine*. Fitzpatrick, T.B., et al.(eds.), 4th ed., New York, McGraw Hill, Inc., 137:1689–1717.

[15] Philips, C.L., Combs, S.B. and Pinnell, S.R.(August 1994) Effects of ascorbic acid on proliferation and collagen synthesis in relation to the donor age of human dermal fibroblasts. *J. of Invest. Dermatol.* 103:228–232.

[16] Rietschel, R.L. and Fowler, J.F., Jr. (1995) *Fisher's Contact Dermatitis*, 4th ed., Baltimore, Williams & Wilkins, 973–1055.

[17] Sheretz, E.F. and Goldsmith, L.A. (1991) Nutritional influences on the skin. In *Physiology, Biochemistry, and Molecular Biology of the Skin*. Goldsmith, L.A. (ed.), New York, Oxford University Press, 49:1315–1328.

[18] Van Scott, E.J. and Yu, R.J. (1974) Control of keratinization with alpha-hydroxy acids and related compounds: I. Topical treatment of ichthyotic disorders. *Arch Dermatol.* 110:586–590.

[19] Wattenberg, L.W. (1985) Chemoprevention of cancer. *Cancer Res.* 45, 1–8.

# About the Author

Ligaya H. Buchbinder, M.D. was born in the town of Pavia, Iloilo in the Philippines. From the age of five, she knew that she wanted to be a doctor. She graduated from elementary school as the valedictorian of her class. After graduation, she travelled at the age of 12 away from her family to Manila (an hour away by airplane) to start high school as a recipient of the highly coveted Philippine Science High School Scholarship. This is awarded through a competitive exam to the top 100 students in the entire nation. After high school graduation, she again received the National Science Development Board Scholarship Award for her pre-medical education. She then proceeded to study to be a doctor of medicine where she met her husband Charles Buchbinder, also a physician.

They moved to New York City to finish their last year of medical school and then to Cincinnati, Ohio to do residency in Dermatology at the University of Cincinnati. They finally settled in Boca Raton, Florida to start their private practice in Dermatology and to raise their family.

Dr. Ligaya Buchbinder has published in medical journals and has served as President of the Palm Beach.Society for Dermatology and Cutaneous Surgery. She is also a member of the American Academy of Dermatology and the American Society for Dermatologic Surgery. Aside from her successful private practice in dermatology, Dr. Buchbinder is also an inventor and has patented the Eyebrow Revolution™ which she has manufactured and marketed through several outlets including television. She is presently working on another revolutionary invention.

Dr. Buchbinder is a woman of many talents and is able to balance her career, family with two young children, hobbies (water-skiing, horseback riding, tennis, windsurfing, cooking, painting, gardening, designing), business entrepreneurship, exercise (daily practice of hatha yoga), and world travel.

As she is writing this book, she is expanding her medical practice and entrepreneurial business at the same time. She sustains a sharp focus over simultaneous projects and turns out clear, solid, and superb outcomes. She is truly capable of thinking, listening, creating, and accomplishing several things at the same time to her very best and fullest energy. This is her utmost talent.

Aside from all her talents, she is a woman with a big heart and outstanding personality. She is truly loved and admired by her patients, friends, and family. You certainly will have a taste of her smart, warm, relaxed, focused, empirical, and practical style as you read this book.

# Index

## A

acne, 6, 7
  causes, 9
  common treatments, 10–11
  cystic, 10, 13
  diet, relationship between, 10
  hair products, relationship between, 106
  hormonal correlation, 11
  make-up application, 133
  premenstrual flare-ups, 12
  scarring, 10
  skin care regimin, 10, 11, 12–13
  whiteheads, 17, 18
acyclovir, 44, 51
adapalene, 10, 20
AHA. *see* alpha hydroxy acids
allergic reactions
  delayed, 6
  immediate, 6
  irritant, 6, 7

alopecia areata, 93–94
alpha hydroxy acids, 6–7, 10, 16, 17, 18, 19, 20, 122, 135, 136
  common ingredients, 18, 127–128
  skin exfoliation, 7
alpha tocopherol. *see* vitamin E
anagen, 87
androgen hormones, 11
antibiotics, 10, 102
  acne treatment, 12, 13
  ointments, 82
  yeast infections, link to, 73, 74
antifungal creams, 70
antihistamines, 38, 48
Aquanil® Lotion, 11, 121, 123
ascorbic acid, 10, 16, 17. *see* vitamin C creams
ascorbyl palmitate, 12, 20
astringent, 136
athlete's foot, 69–71

hydrocortisone cream, 36, 66
  dandruff, use as treatment
      for, 98, 99
hydroquinone, 54, 55

# I

idiopathic guttate
      hypomelanosis, 55
impetigo, 81–83
ingrown hair
  bacterial infection risk, 102
  causes, 101
  shaving tips, 101–102
  symptoms, 101
itching, 136–137
  bug bites. *see* bug bites
  chickenpox. *see* chickenpox
  common treatments, 37
  over-the-counter remedies,
      37
  scratching, 35
  underlying causes,
      importance of
      diagnosis, 36
IvyBlock®, 20

# J

Jessner's solution, 123, 124
jock itch, 69–71

# K

kojic acid, 55
Kwell®, 104

# L

lactic acid, 18, 39, 40
Lamisil®, 115
lanocaine, 36, 50
lanolin, 5, 6, 33, 122
lanugo hair, 88
L-ascorbic acid, 20
laser
  common types used, 141
  definition, 140
  surgery, 18
    argon, 79
lentigines. *see* freckles
levodopa, link to hair loss, 95
lice
  diagnosis, 103
  head, 103–104
  infestation areas, 103
  pubic, 103–104
  spread, 104
  treatments, 104
Ligaya® Eyebrow Revolution,
      95, 109
liposuction, 141–142
liquid nitrogen, 78
liver spots, 54
L-lysine, as canker sore
      treatment, 44–45

# M

make-up. *see* cosmetics
malnourishment, link to
      chronic yeast
      infections, 75

vitamin deficiencies. *see*
        nutritional
        deficiencies
vitamin E, 5, 129–130
vitiligo, 55

# W

warts
    affected areas, 39
    causes, 39
    length of treatment, 40–41
    methods of spreading, 39
    treatment, 39–40
        over-the-counter
            remedies, 40
        tape, occlusive, 40
water, importance to skin
        health, 10, 11
waxing (hair), 95, 96, 102, 108
whiteheads. *see* acne

witch hazel, 37
wrinkles
    cosmetic procedures, 18–19
    crow's feet, 15
    cultural acceptance, 15
    eye area, 7
    facial expression, 15
    prevention, 19
    sunbathing, 15
    sun damage, 15

# Y

yeast infections, 73–75
yoga, 16
yogurt, for yeast infections,
        74–75

# Z

Zovirax®, 44